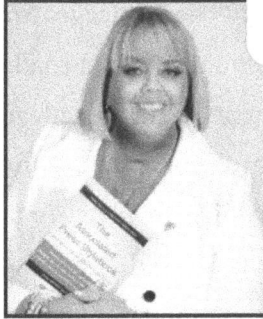

In 2004, **Janet Sutherland** suffered from a ruptured brain aneurysm that left her blind and paralyzed. She has now fully recovered and has turned her health trauma into a career by lobbying and fundraising for the Brain Aneurysm Foundation.

Sutherland's name may be familiar; she was on Chicago's airwaves in the 1990's. She is a former Chicago radio reporter where she was heard covering Supreme Court cases, Illinois legislation, health news and prison stories on WMAQ, WLS, WGN, KMOX, UPI Radio and 75 plus radio stations on the Illinois and Wisconsin Radio Networks. As a result of covering breaking news stories; the deadly Plainfield/Lemont Tornado, Joliet Correctional prison escape, her newsroom was the recipient of AP awards. While a journalist Sutherland's news stories were distributed on ABC News, AP and UPI wire services and aired on at least 75 radio stations in the Midwest. She has also written and produced cable television public affairs programs. She was also a feature freelance writer for The Daily Herald and a sports stringer for The Chicago Sun Times. Sutherland worked with the Illinois News Broadcaster's Association in speaking engagements at local colleges. She also served on the Junior Board of the Museum of Broadcast Communications which involved organizing "The Salute to Larry King." She has worked in marketing in cable television and has syndicated national radio shows and news networks including CNN, CBS and Fox.

That day, March 22, 2004, friends and family sat at Janet's bedside, she was given 3 percent chance to live. For weeks as co-workers, raised money for her family and joined her battle and prayed she would survive. After spending years in rehabilitation, Sutherland wrote two bills to promote the disease around the Midwest, she now speaks regularly on Chicago radio stations and on TV about her brain aneurysm experience.

JANET SUTHERLAND-MADDEN

NOSE
OVER
TOES

ECKHARTZ
PRESS

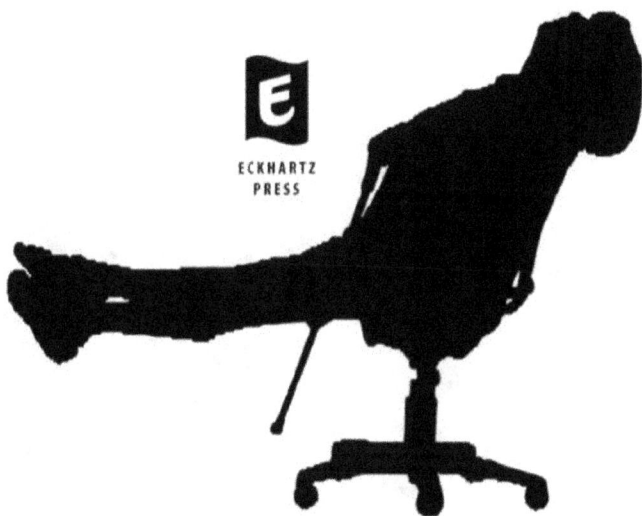

This book is dedicated to my family, for their endless support and untellable affection. I am forever grateful. To my husband Kevin: for your love, kindness, and devotion. The Brain Aneurysm Foundation, for their invaluable information for survivors and unending medical research, has been extraordinary for my family, friends and survivors. Also, to all the neurosurgeons, neurologists, nurses, physical therapists, retina specialists, neuroradiologists and first responders: my cup runneth over because of the lifesaving care given to me. It is also important to recognize and honor those who did not survive a brain aneurysm.

On Monday, June 25, 2018, my father lost his battle with bladder cancer. He worked with me on this book until his last breath. Dad leaves behind wonderful memories of his incredible generosity, strength, and love. He lived a life committed to his family and to community service. I hope this book ensures that my father's legacy of helping others lives on.

Thank you, Dad, for carrying a pen and notepad in your shirt pocket; without you, this book wouldn't have been written.

Donald Ripley Sutherland
July 28, 1932 - June 25, 2018
Rest in Peace. You will never be forgotten.

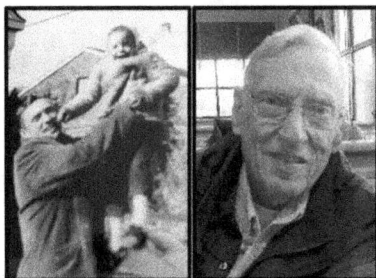

TABLE OF CONTENTS

FOREWORD

By Donald R. Sutherland

I kept a journal of Janet's ordeal in order to record both the events and her treatment. One of the most helpful comments a doctor made to us was this: "Don't look for progress day by day, but week by week." It's an understatement to say that we all learned patience. We are hoping this book will be an educational story and an inspirational piece to teach people how to survive.

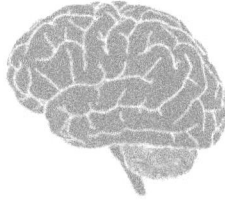

CHAPTER 1

911

I tugged at the wheels of my wheelchair, tears streaming down my face. I couldn't find my room. I was in a hospital, but I didn't even know what city I was in. Some onlookers, fellow patients, were calling out directions as I navigated the stark hallway. "Keep going, you're getting close." I was so confused. How could I have ended up this way: blind, paralyzed, and in a wheelchair?

It all started on the evening of March 22, 2004. In addition to battling a sinus infection, I'd been suffering from a constant headache for months, and I was taking four aspirin daily. My co-workers at WTVN radio in Columbus, Ohio continually raised their concerns about my aspirin and antibiotic intake. Being focused on the more recent sinus infection and not my constant headache or strange vision change, I left my office as usual that day. I needed to get home to take my dog, Bogie, for a walk. Upon arriving at my apartment, my headache magnified exponentially, unlike anything I had experienced before: it felt like my ears were going to pop off. I immediately called my mom in Glen Ellyn, Illinois, because I figured if I was going to die, I should say goodbye. She told me to get to an emergency room. I called 911, crying hysterically, "I have the biggest headache on the planet. I need help!" Then I collapsed on my kitchen floor. I have no memory of the rest of that day. The following are my father's notes of what happened.

After dinner, at about 6:20 pm on Monday, March 22, 2004, Janet called home before calling 911. The medics arrived four minutes later and found her unconscious, with Bogie sitting next to her. Fortunately, she had left the door open so they were able to get in and quickly move her into an ambulance for the drive to Doctors West Hospital.

The ER doctor gave me a three percent chance of living and had me transferred to a trauma hospital. Dr. Joseph Shehadi at Columbus' Grant Medical Center described my initial condition as "at death's door"; I had suffered a ruptured brain aneurysm. Before my emergency brain surgery, he whispered to me to "be brave." Although I was unconscious at the time, weeks later I remembered hearing him say that. I underwent a six-hour operation, during which a metal clip was placed in my brain to stop the bleeding.

While I lay unconscious in the hospital my parents were racing from their home in Glen Ellyn to be by my side, my brother having arranged their airline tickets. As my parents raced to the gate to catch the plane, my dad placed a call to my Aunt Dot, his sister. He frantically told her what had happened and said, "We can't lose Janet, we just can't lose her." Aunt Dot told my dad, "We just need to pray, that's all we can do." Calls were placed to prayer chains as far as Africa for me. My Glenbard West High School friends started an email chain which updated everyone on my condition. From what I was told, old friends caught up during the emails. Go figure - I was always the party planner and tended to bring everyone together; after all, I did plan a couple high school reunions.

My father continued his journal:

We thought it was too late to catch a plane out of O'Hare but rushed to get our things together in hopes we could. Our neighbor, Darrell Holsteen, drove us to O'Hare where we caught the last American flight to Columbus. The plane was held 15 minutes so we could make it. Run we did; Marie twisted her knee and stretched a ligament as we raced through the airport to the gate, but we made it!

Dr. William Frazier at Doctors West Hospital said Janet has suffered a massive blood spill from a burst aneurysm on the right side of her brain above the right ear; the chances of her surviving are only 50 percent. If she survives, she could suffer paralysis or worse. She has undergone a CAT scan that revealed no information other than large quantities of spilled blood. It is necessary for her to undergo an angiogram, which is why she has been moved to Grant Medical Center in downtown Columbus.

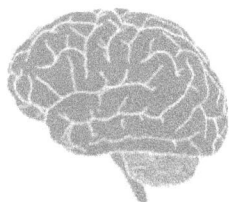

CHAPTER 2

Shopping in my Dreams

I was in a coma for three weeks. My father sat at my bedside every night, holding my hand and saying repeatedly, "Everything will be okay." He read my favorite children's stories to me.

During that time, I dreamed I was back in Chicago shopping along Michigan Avenue at the Louis Vuitton store. I was the fictional character Carrie Bradshaw from the HBO show *Sex and The City*. Back when I worked for radio syndicator Westwood One, I would sometimes grab my Gucci sunglasses and my only Louis Vuitton purse and strut up and down Michigan Avenue on half-inch heels. I'd prance around a construction area along the sidewalk thinking, "I am the shizzle," all the while channeling my inner Carrie Bradshaw. On one such occasion, while strutting and clutching my Louis Vuitton, I took a tumble right there on the sidewalk. Was I hurt? Who cares, I had my Louis. I popped up, turned around, and traipsed boldly back to work.

So that's why I was shopping along Michigan Avenue while in my coma. I was not just fighting for my life: I was fighting for the fabulous future I once had. I was determined to battle whatever I had to, in order to stay alive.

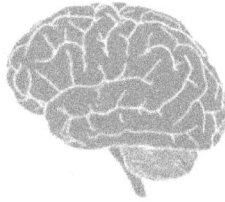

CHAPTER 3

What Did I Miss?

This was not at all in my plans. I was thirty-eight years old and had moved to Columbus, Ohio just two years earlier to be with a guy who I thought offered a serious relationship. I had always fantasized about getting married in my twenties, being pregnant in Glen Ellyn, and living in a lovely home with a white picket fence. I would have my journalism career behind me after a short stint in New York City at the "network," and then I would be a "Martha Stewart" sexy wife. But instead, now I was on prayer lists across the country. When I woke up, I learned that Julia Roberts was pregnant with twins, J Lo had gotten married, and Easter had already happened. I missed out on a lot of chocolate bunnies. Yes, I felt really ripped off!

However, a lot went on during those three weeks other than the pop culture that I had missed. Katie, my first friend in Ohio who was with me in the ER, snuck into a local Catholic church and scooped up some holy water which she delivered to me in the ICU. She and my mom placed cool washcloths on my head. Katie also promised God she would give me her Louis Vuitton purse if I lived.

When I finally woke up I asked my friends in the news business, "What did I miss?" You can't get the reporter out of me since that had been my whole life. I was one of the first female sports reporters for the Glen Ellyn Newspapers. I really enjoyed talking and telling stories, and that's how I landed in radio news. I did a brief stint in TV news as an intern. I won an award for breaking a big story. I knew after I woke up and slowly heard the stats about brain aneurysms that this is a story that has been shamefully overlooked. So, at the urging of my reporter friends and other brain aneurysm survivors, I am writing this book.

I owe my father a great deal; he kept an amazingly detailed journal of my battle for survival and recovery. Getting your life back to normal can be done. You can live with metal in your head. You can survive with the prospect of another brain aneurysm, once you continue to get screened. You are not alone. You can take control of your health with a great team of doctors: general practitioners, neurologists, neurosurgeons, and retina specialist.

There are many journeys that make up the big hurdle called life. I began to realize this while wheeling down the hallway in the hospital. Everything I had experienced up to that point would help me overcome the daunting task of getting my life back: walking, seeing, and functioning as a normal human being with or without handicaps. That is what this book is about. I did get a Louis Vuitton purse from Katie. While I don't encourage bargaining with God, it was a funny and sweet gesture from my great friend.

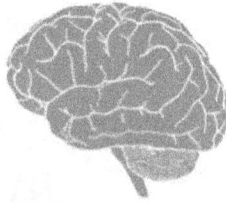

CHAPTER 4

Reporting

My parents, Don and Marie Sutherland, received a call from an Episcopal-based adoption agency in Maryland on the day I was born. They were told to expect a strawberry-blonde baby girl. They were both well-educated, committed, and ready for adoption and any accompanying challenges. Growing up, I was teased about being adopted. To make matters worse, I was in the slower math classes and had special tutors. Reading and writing were also difficult because I had a learning disability. The teachers told my parents that I would "never read or write and probably not amount to much of a student." However, my parents made sure I received special tutoring, and I was determined to prove those teachers wrong big time.

My beautiful mother's large, loving family emigrated to America from Greece. Of Scottish lineage, my father comes from the upper crust. His family members are at home in the accounting world and are very success-driven. I don't look Greek at all, and I still can barely balance my checkbook. Luckily, I do look a bit Scottish. One thing is for sure; it's amazing that I graduated from college, which made both the Sutherland and Constanitopolispapavasolopolis (changed to Panor at Ellis Island) families proud.

After graduating with a degree in Communication Media from St. Norbert College, I realized a six-figure reporter's job was not going to happen right away. I would eventually pursue my dream job as a radio reporter in Chicago, but in the meantime, I worked for free at WFXW-AM in Geneva, Illinois. I worked the Sunday morning shift, running religious songs at the wrong speed and engineering a religious show with "Brother Wes." Brother Wes would stride into the studio followed by his wife, whom he referred to as "Mother." She sat in the corner of the studio, reading her Bible with her lips pressed together. When Brother Wes preached, he was so loud that I had to turn his mic down very low. He had no problem using the microphone sometime later to criticize the radio management.

Eventually, I did get paid for the Sunday morning stint and for reading news headlines, as needed. The radio station's signal was so weak that during the holidays my family had to drive around the block of the station to hear me. I did take some heat from them for saying, "I'm outta here," as I signed off from my show. I guess that wasn't appropriate during my "God Squad" show. This was my problem in news and the media. I found so much humor in just about everything that I could hardly behave while covering anything from a school board meeting to an execution.

Job after suburban job, I finally made it to the city when I was hired at the Illinois radio network as Chicago bureau chief, at the Thompson Center. I sat in the press room with the Chicago Sun Times, the Chicago Tribune, City News, and others like UPI and AP. Trying to be a hotshot in this room of big guns, I accepted invitations from the Illinois Department of Corrections to be a media witness of executions. As a female reporter, I witnessed more executions than most. I accepted these emotionally difficult assignments to prove my moxie as a journalist.

In the Thompson Center pressroom, I stood out as the only radio reporter. It also helped that my hair was a different shade of red every few months; the governor's press secretary told my boss he never knew what color my hair was going to be when he saw me. I was surprised at how all the reporters spoke into the phone with their hands covering their mouths, protecting the information they passed on to their editors. I had the golden ticket: a fax machine which helped me break news quicker than everyone else. It also meant that a big part of my job, other than getting the story and meeting the deadline, involved scrambling around for fax paper and batteries for my tape deck. Needless to say, radio reporting was quite underrated at the time.

There were many executions in Illinois in the early 90s; it seemed like that was the focus of my work. We maintained a list of those executed and what their last meals were. One particularly notable execution was that of John Wayne Gacy. When he requested a Diet Coke, *Inside Edition* started a furor during the press briefing in the media tent. Why a Diet Coke rather than, say, a milkshake? It seemed ridiculous to me, and I thought, Enough! I needed a new career, away from reporting.

My parents begged me to stay at the network until after the 1996 Democratic National Convention, which I did. It was an amazing experience. I ran into NBC journalist Tim Russert on the convention floor. He was holding a reporter's notebook and actually doing the leg-work. Every reporter in politics looked up to him; he was a network star who could have had one of his interns doing that work. Russert died in 2008 of a heart attack while covering a story. My most popular story with the 50-plus radio stations was how many pounds of food the media consumed in the media tent during the 1996 convention. The media food tent served Chicago's finest foods like Eli's cheesecake on a stick. I remember standing behind Ed Bradley from CBS News and Tabatha Soren from MTV, stupidly star struck.

Although my reporting career is over, I am still great friends with many people from that time. The fact that many are now a permanent fixture in my life is due to one person, Congressman Mel Reynolds. Representative Reynolds was convicted of having sex with an underage former campaign worker and then trying to thwart the investigation. The trial lasted a month and was full of colorful testimony. Reporters from UPI, AP the *Chicago Tribune, Chicago Sun Times,* CNN, and all the local TV stations and wire services spent 12 hour days together to get in front of the line at the courthouse so we could get a good seat at the trial. Testimony was salacious. I actually ate off of the food truck and tried not to get kicked out of the courtroom when the naughty testimony started detailing the sexual relationship the Congressman, was accused of having with an underage campaign worker. Some of the testimony included lewd details involving peach panties which caught headlines the next day.

The press corps waited in line to get a seat in the courtroom as early as 5 a.m. One of the TV reporters wrote a limerick about some of the testimony. To win over some of the hard-core, veteran print reporters in the courthouse pressroom, I baked cookies for them. I worked 11-plus hours pushing my mic through the media crowd, trying to get a great sound bite and loving every minute of it. One of the TV reporters would complain that I was always in their shot.

I snickered thinking, Yea that's my point, just as long as my boss sees me doing my job, ha!

On one of the last days of the trial, I sat with some other female reporters behind a WGN TV reporter. We must have been rather punchy, because she turned around and said, "You girls must have low blood sugar," and she handed us candy. We probably did have low blood sugar; we were so broke, we ate from the food trucks in front of the courthouse. Our pitiful salaries barely paid for our parking. Mel Reynolds' last word to all of us in the media was, "Get out of my way or I'll take you down," as he walked off to the courthouse to surrender himself to serve his sentence.

Throughout the trial, we journalists spent so much time together we ended up meeting at The Billy Goat Tavern, a famous bar that was parodied on Saturday Night Live: "Cheeseburger, cheeseburger, cheeseburger, cheeseburger!" Mike Royko, the notoriously grumpy columnist for the *Chicago Tribune*, was well known for showing up at the drinking hole and peeing outside of the bar, making no excuses. Yep, the joint was a dump, like a roughed-up *Cheers*, but you really felt like you were part of the tough, old Chicago journalist group. I was starstruck, starving and yearning for sleep, and I felt like I needed a manicure. Well at least I survived a rough trial and made it to "The Goat." I was so sorry to see the trial end. One thing was for sure: another Illinois politician will more than likely go to trial for something else, but I made great friends and learned some good reporting techniques.

I served my time as a reporter: 10 years in Chicago. Two of my reporter friends from that time participated in my wedding: one shared a reading and another sang. I am lucky enough to still have my memory, so I can tell this story.

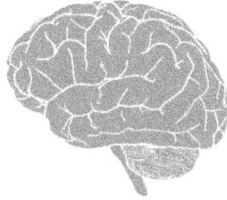

CHAPTER 5

Learn From Yesterday and Focus on Tomorrow

Right before my brain aneurysm ruptured, the United States began the war with Iraq and eventually murdered Saddam Hussein's sons. At that time, I worked at a radio station in Columbus, Ohio, as a member of the sales staff. My co-workers and I huddled in front of the TV, conflicted about the war and debating whether it was the right move for our country.

Upon waking from my coma, I thought I was in that war. Not only was I blind and partially paralyzed, I was greatly confused. Even worse, I was tied down by my hands and feet. This was to prevent me from attempting to get out of bed. Doctors explained to my parents that my brain was trying to put things back together, but I was behaving as though I was a prisoner in the Iraq war. This I remember in particular: when the pulse oximeter would go off, I would try to sit up in the bed and bend toward my feet, my hands folded in prayer. I really did think it was a call to prayer and that I was in an Iraqi prison. The fact that I was tied down confirmed to me that I was in an Iraqi prison. I thought my neurosurgeon Dr. Joseph Shehadi was actually Saddam Hussein.

It probably didn't help that the hospital building next to mine was being imploded for new building construction. In my blind state, I could see only shadows. A trache in my throat made it very difficult for me to speak. My handwriting had always been horrible but the only way I could communicate was to write my thoughts; however, no one could read what I wrote. So here is the picture: I am in an Iraqi prison camp, tied up, can't speak, no one can read my handwriting, and there's lots of explosive noises nearby. So, I was convinced I was losing my mind. My dad journaled my frustration from his vantage point:

April 17 - She is upset now that she has realized the extent of her injury and that she is not able to move her left side or talk. She wants the trachea out but this can't be done while she is on blood thinners. Doctors will put in a different trachea valve.

She is very anxious and wants to get out. When upset, blood pressure goes up to 170 and beyond and heart rate goes from 99 to 124.

She is able to squeeze my finger with her left hand and her strength is expected to improve. When she tried to sit up, she was dizzy; she's still on an antibiotic for fever and anti-depressants. She does not like being dependent, particularly when friends visit, and this is a big source of her agitation.

April 21 – Janet has difficulty talking and a correct valve for the trache tube has not been found. Dillusional can cause forgetfulness and difficulty in piecing words together; sufferers are not always able to speak in complete sentences; occasionally, they can only manage fragments. When asked to read a sign that gave the name of the unit where she was staying, she whispered, "Free chocolate ice cream for Janet," indicating that dillusional is not a problem and her sense of humor is alive. Things are looking up. Later in the day she swung her left leg over the side of the bed; this was a first. Yesterday she squeezed someone with her left hand, indicating that the nerves are beginning to heal and some of her strength is returning. Although she needed a sedative and an antibiotic in the afternoon to fight an infection, her temperature was down to 99 degrees.

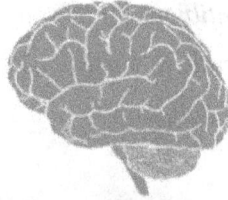

CHAPTER 6

My Big Secret

What my family was not aware of was that I was blind when I awoke from my coma; I could perceive only shadows. I did everything I could do to hide this. Even though I was delusional regarding where I was, at the same time I didn't want my blindness to be discovered. I didn't want to cause my parents more grief, and I was trying to process how I would deal with blindness. For instance, when the staff asked me to read a sign, I thought I would be clever and said, "Free ice cream for everyone." It worked! People laughed, and I bought myself more time. I used my sense of smell to remember the different nurses and technicians who tended to me. "Darn this is gonna be tough to avoid," I was thinking, "But as long as I don't have to read an eye chart, I will be good." I couldn't bear further upsetting my family; they had come all the way from Chicago to be with me.

Incidentally, for some time I thought I was in Chicago and didn't realize Columbus even had any hospitals; more evidence of the big confusion going on in my head! And where was my dog Bogie? I didn't understand why no one was speaking about him, but I didn't dwell on that fact; I really couldn't think about anything for very long. I could barely handle the functions of each day. My dad journaled about Bogie:

April 22 – Staff are still trying to find a valve to fit the trache tube to help Janet speak more easily. She remains on a sedative to control agitation but was able to sit up twice during the day. She has hallucinations, imagining that the dog across the street attacked Bogie, but, since that did nearly happen, it did not seem to be a big stretch from reality. In any event, her physical and speech therapists say they are pleased with her progress.

At this point in my recovery, I figured I had suffered a stroke. When my parents tried to explain to me by saying "an ANNNEEUUURYYYYYYYYYYYSSSSSSSSMMM," I thought, "What do they think, I'm an idiot? Yea I had a stroke; what the heck is an aneurysm? Geesh what are they talking about!"

My emotional state was extremely unstable. When my friends came by, I totally lost my filter and acted as if I had turned into a standup comedian, blurting out quite inappropriate words. One time I even referred to a nurse as a cow. I didn't mean to be disrespectful, but my vision made it difficult to see things correctly. My vision had returned to the point that I did have some peripheral vision. But delusions continued to creep back on occasion. At one point, I was convinced that there were snipers in the hospital parking garage, aiming at my family. This was a difficult time for my parents, according to my dad's journal.

April 23 – Janet joked and was in a good mood. Friends visited and when she was told that she was in a hospital, she said, "Stop treating me like I'm a two-year old." She had therapy even though it was Saturday. A new trache tube has been ordered but she can talk using the old one even though it is plugged. She talked to a girlfriend about clients and contracts at work, but she switches from reality to fantasy without changing gears. Staff at the hospital think she is doing amazingly well considering what she has been through. Her strength in her left hand has increased and she can squeeze it amazingly well. She tried to get out of bed using her right leg and staff had to restrain it; whereupon, she started to use her left leg, paralyzed by the aneurysm, to propel herself out of bed. When this leg had to be restrained, she resisted with a lot of pressure.

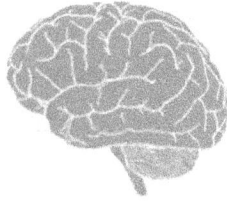

CHAPTER 7

Will I Ever Be My "Old Self" Again?

My recovery was bumpy, but everyone knew I was on the way back to my old self when I flipped off a nurse in the hospital. The offensive gesture was a positive sign to my friends and family that I was back to my usual feisty self. Surprisingly, even my dad was excited that I gave someone the finger. His journal describes the slow healing progress.

April 24 – Janet seems more alert today. She greeted her morning nurse with a smile and the "middle finger" salute, telling everybody that she was not happy where she was. She wants a female nurse and to be able to get out of bed and sit in a chair. He responded that her "spirit" was a good sign.

I was completely confused about what hospital I was in because I never knew Columbus, Ohio had any notable hospitals. I had been in a coma for three weeks following brain surgery. In medical lingo, it is called a craniotomy. I struggled greatly with fatigue. Because my core muscles had weakened, I could barely sit up in a wheelchair. Much of the time, I had no idea what was going on around me. My dad includes this in his journal. I was able to speak more by this time, at least.

April 25 – Janet rested most of the day, but she did ask about Bogie and we told her that he was fine. She has not been told about his ruptured disc and the unsuccessful surgery that left him unable to walk. She must be told, but we are waiting for all of us to be together before telling her. We can't keep putting this off. We have to tell her soon.

April 26 – Janet talked a lot and joked with staff. She had one and one half hours of speech and occupational therapy. Doctors and staff are planning to move her to Grant South in one week.

The lease on Janet's apartment expires on Friday but it can be extended six months. Another weekly disability check came in the mail. Janet is still suffering hallucinations and Bogie has become incontinent. This was a bit of a down day.

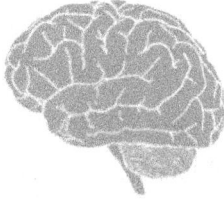

CHAPTER 8

Bogie

My illness wasn't just hell for me; it was also very hard on my family. I was clueless as to what was going on. My Dad's journal helps piece it together for me:

April 28 - Staff say that it is hard to make a complete diagnosis of her condition because she is compensating to meet the restrictions caused by the aneurysm. She has some blood in her lungs, but staff will be able to suction it out. The blood may be the result of coughing. Janet had a two-hour physical therapy session this morning and took a one and a half hour nap in the afternoon. She ate a peanut butter sandwich for lunch and is able to speak easier with the new trachea valve. The psychologist says that we have to level with her about Bogie's ruptured disc and paralysis in a calm and loving manner. He has had a lot of scars and is getting increasingly depressed. She must know his condition is bad and will not get better.

Though my vision had somewhat improved, I was still legally blind. My left side was still completely paralyzed. I was aware that my family was worried about me, and I felt vaguely and continually unsettled. My family and friends tried to take care of Bogie: they visited him at my apartment and even at the vet's office. Once, they brought Bogie to visit me in the hospital. He sat briefly on my bed in a crate, and I knew that my dog was very sick. My little buddy, who had guarded me on the kitchen floor while my brain was bleeding, was, like me, now unable to walk. He needed me, and I couldn't be there for him.

When I turned six years old, my dad bought me a dog. My parents had been told that a corgi was the best kind of dog for children, and so they brought Corky into our family. She was a retired world champion and very patient: she let me put my ballet tutu on her head and parade her around in a wagon all dressed up. She never growled or looked unhappy. Corky was quite dignified and tolerant of the nonsense we put her through.

When I was grown and began looking to get a dog, Corky was my standard. I combed through the pet section of the *Chicago Sun Times* while I sat in the pressroom on breaks. I could not imagine I would ever find another sweet corgi, but life was lonely without a pooch. Finally, one afternoon, there was an ad for a corgi living on a farm way out in the country. I was so broke that I could barely afford the dog, but my brother agreed to give me the money. I was very skeptical that this corgi would really be in good health and suitable, but my mom and I drove out to see him anyway. When we pulled up to the farm, there was a pen full of goats and chickens and a skinny little corgi barking at us. I thought, No wonder he's hungry! All of the livestock are eating his food. I knocked on the farmhouse door. The woman who answered was pregnant, like any-moment pregnant, and her husband, wearing a wife-beater shirt, came out to discuss the dog whose name was Bogie. The woman said she had rescued him from a kill shelter but didn't have time for him now. When she let Bogie out of the pen, he ran around on the grass. When I called him, he ran into my arms and we were buddies immediately. He was tan and white with just a stub of a tail. Mom and I fell in love with him. Mr. Boo, my cat, hated him, so I gave the cat to my parents and Bogie made himself at home.

Our network studios were in a dog-friendly building so Bogie would come to work with me every day. The radio station owners kept a jar of dog treats for my pooch, but when I'd let Bogie sit in my anchor chair, that was another story. The morning anchor would know Bogie was visiting because Bogie's fur was all over the chair and I would get an angry call asking, "Was Bogie here over the weekend?" I would say Yes but just briefly. I wonder who else he thought would leave white fur everywhere. The sports reporter at the station would beg to babysit Bogie some weekends. I had to keep turning him down, because I would have missed Bogie. He really was quite a celebrity. One of the managers kept teasing me about how big Bogie's head was, with all the attention Bogie was getting at work. He even would sit in the studio with me when I anchored the news. It was odd: Bogie seemed to know to be quiet when I was on the air. He was a good dog.

Like most little dogs, Bogie thought he was a big dog in a little dog's body. I took him to the dog park in Chicago where he proceeded to nip a big dog and I was yelled at and barred from going back I had no idea he was so aggressive, but it turned out that Bogie was very protective of me and a great watchdog. Once, when I was doing a weekend shift, there was an attempted break-in and Bogie scared away the burglar while I was on the air. But he also did get into trouble. The stupidest thing he ever did was attack an Akita, a large ferocious dog who didn't like being bitten in the chest. I think Bogie was trying to prove who was boss but it cost him a piece of his ear and required him to wear a cone for a week. He walked around with one ear taped down and the other ear sticking up, looking like an airplane with a propeller missing. People continued to ask me, "Does he have the other ear?" (So he's cute but dumb.)

Our first Christmas, Bogie peed on the baby Jesus in my crèche, and he ate all the chocolate Christmas cookies. He went everywhere with me; we traveled together and shared car rides to the store and picked out his treats at the pet store. When we moved to different homes, it was always comforting that Bogie was with me; he was family. My neighbors always knew Bogie; they would call out and greet him when we'd go for walks. I loved sharing life with him. Remembering some of these things while I stayed in the hospital made me miss Bogie all the more.

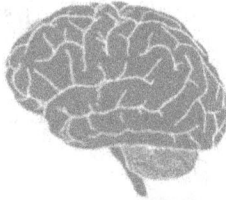

CHAPTER 9

More Obstacles (Or Blessings)

April 29 - Very agitated in the morning, Janet was given medication that made her very sleepy. Yesterday she had been able to move her left arm horizontally but today she was able to move it vertically against gravity for the first time. Tomorrow we are to meet with staff to see if Janet can stay at Select Special Hospital for an extra week past the regularly assigned two weeks. She is not ready to go to Grant South Hospital for intensive occupational therapy and in cases where this happens, the patient is usually sent to a skilled nursing facility where those with chronic conditions are not expected to get better. This would be a step down for Janet; rather than inspirational, it would only be depressive. We want her to stay at Special Select for an extra week of special care in hope that she will be able to go to Grant South the week after that.

To get into Grant South, she has to be able to handle 3 hours of occupational therapy per day. Unfortunately, if she has to go to either of these nursing facilities, she will not receive occupational training. This leaves us with the only alternative of convincing the Patient Advocate that an extra week is the correct course of action; then persuading her to convince United Health Care of the same thing. Fortunately, a team of three therapists, a nurse, a psychologist, and a case manager reviewed Janet's case and decided that an extra week at Special Select was the best course of action. With their recommendation, approval by the insurance company is expected. This is a blessing. Our visits to two nursing care facilities revealed that they would not be places where Janet could interact positively with others aspiring to get out and re-enter normal life on the outside. These residents were older patients whose age and handicap would likely not permit them to leave a nursing home.

My doctors and family finally figured out that I was hiding my lack of vision from them. I think my method of eating may have first clued them in: I once put my hand in the chocolate mousse! It may seem funny, but I love to eat dessert, not wear it! My co-workers were great, visiting me in the hospital and raising money to help my family while they stayed in my apartment. I guess some of my friends figured out I couldn't see according to my Dad's journal.

April 30 – Janet has begun eating with a fork; she also sat up for 5 hours and had 1 1/2 hours of therapy. These are positive signs; however, there are indications she has vision problems. At this point, there is no way to determine the extent of the damage to her sight. Howard, her colleague at the office, came to visit and she told him that it was scary being in the hospital, unable to see and not knowing what was going on. She also had scary feelings that she did not know her own mind.

My radio news experience and just all-around big talker personality were coming back to haunt me. I could not stop talking even though I was encouraged to. Many who know me would not be surprised that I talked more than the nurses and doctors preferred. I talked one day so much that my trache started to bleed. This was actually worse than not being able to walk freely. I had a lot of questions and needed to know what exactly had happened to me. This was affecting my healing process according to my Dad's journal.

May 1 - Janet is still experiencing fears and times of great sleepiness; the speech therapist told her not to try to talk but just relax, since her strength is low and she is breathing a 30 percent mixture of oxygen. She is off the anxiety medication during the day; it is necessary only at night.

Friends came by to visit and we were planning to tell her about Bogie's ruptured disc that has paralyzed his hindquarters. He is very sad and there is nothing that can be done to help him except to buy a two-wheeled cart to put his rear feet in so he does not have to drag them. Since Janet is extremely tired and not able to talk because of the trachea situation, we've decided to delay telling her about Bogie's injury.

I remember being so hungry because I couldn't see my food and was afraid the trache was going to cause me to choke on my food. The whole healing process was humiliating: I wore a catheter, diapers, and basically a bib when I ate. Who was this inept woman in a hospital bed? I used to be a fearless reporter who cops would call and tip off on stories. And when I was with my girlfriends, I wore glamorous rhinestone earrings, fur coats and tall, shiny, black boots. I would risk frostbite in Chicago to make sure I looked fabulous. Now I was drooling and wearing diapers. What a nightmare!! People would walk in and tell me what a miracle I was and how lucky and blessed I should feel. Well, I felt as though I had already lost my life.

My Dad saw everything as a blessing. I thought he was crazy. I couldn't sit straight in the wheelchair and was so tired I would nap in it, slouched halfway down. What a sight I must have been!

May 2 - Janet is able to feed herself when eating salad and many other foods but not when eating cereal; the milk runs down her face and she can't stop it. My brother Mark came by to visit as well as co-workers from Janet's office. It was good for her to see them; they cheered her up.

She is expected to have one more week in Select Specialty (an intense inpatient rehabilitation unit) and then transfer to Grant South (a rehabilitation Hospital), if approved by the insurance company as we expect. If not, she will have to go out to the boondocks to one of the chronic care health facilities that cater to people who are not expected to improve to the point where they can live on her own.

May 8 - I visited Bogie at Avery Hospital. He can walk using the cart that supports his back legs, but the lack of exercise since the injury has left him in a weakened condition. Also, he has refused to eat for several days, not even treats, and he looks very sad. It seems to be only a matter of time before he has to be put to sleep to take him out of his misery. Janet had her blood pressure taken and it was good, 108 over 82. She and I went for a walk this afternoon, she was in the wheelchair and I pushed her out the emergency room door around the building to the front door where we met Dr. Shehadi and Dr. Mahmood who were surprised and happy to see us. I remember that Dr. Mahmood advised us to look for progress on a weekly rather than a daily basis because it is happening at such a slow rate that it can't be noticed at more frequent intervals.

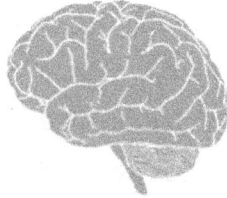

CHAPTER 10

The Iraq War

I continued to think, on occasion, that I was in the middle of the Iraq War, particularly when the staff was taping up the windows and there were loud exploding sounds. Who could blame me?

A moment of local excitement was coming soon, when the O'Rourke Destruction Company was to bring down an old hospital building to make way for the construction of a new building in Grant Medical Center. The event was to be covered on local television, and the mayor and other dignitaries would be on hand when the blasting occurred, and the walls came tumbling down. When this happened, great clouds of smoke arose and the building dropped, just as planned, without disturbing any of the others around it. It was a marvel of modern engineering to be sure, but it convinced me that I was indeed in the middle of the Iraqi War. Thinking back now, I was probably not the only patient on the neurology floor who was totally confused. I can only imagine the chaos this caused for patients and the staff. Personally, I thought for sure that snipers were out to get my parents and friends, and I warned everyone as they left. Some were amused, and I became quite the sideshow of "crazy town." My parents were worried. As if things couldn't get worse, my heart broke the next day, my Dad explains in his journal:

May 9 - We learned that Bogie died in his sleep earlier this morning. One of the interns at the veterinary hospital found him dead when she went up in the morning to check on him. He had stopped eating shortly after the unsuccessful disc surgery had forced him to depend on a cart to support his hind legs as he propelled himself using only his front legs. I remember the depressed look on his face when he saw that this was the condition he was in. It was too much and he decided not to continue living. He stopped eating and died in four days.

Janet is still on Coumadin, antibiotics, and a stomach-coating pill; her blood pressure is 110 over 78. It was a quiet day and she is scheduled to go to Grant South on Monday or Tuesday. We were told there might be a delay because of the implosion bringing down Old Baldwin but this shouldn't be more than a day. Janet was able to move herself in the wheelchair using her left hand as well as her right; this was a big move forward and shows that she is getting back use of her left arm.

May 10 - Janet has taken some steps in therapy; she needs the thinner soled tennis shoes for balance and comfort. Her chest was vacuumed and brought up a white fluid but showed no sign of infection. Her blood pressure was 128 over 82 and temperature was 98.7 degrees. Dr. King removed stitches in her throat that have been a problem. They came out easily and quickly.

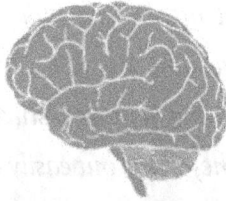

CHAPTER 11

Ready For Boot Camp

May 11 – I went into the hospital in late morning as Janet was having lunch. I thought I would have to help her eat it because of her restricted vision, but she could get the food on her fork when told the hour of the clock where the particular serving was located. She had a good lunch of macaroni, meat, tossed salad, chocolate mouse and milk but was unable to eat all of any portion except the glass of milk. She did well. Janet is ready to go to Grant South except for some paper work processing that will be completed tomorrow. Her sight is now the biggest problem and whether it can be treated. She cannot read and sees mostly shadows. Her arm and leg are beginning to come around. Today she had her leg draped over the side of the bed and someone brought her a soccer ball that she was able to kick. This was a big step forward; she could bend her knee and get her foot on the ball. I left for Chicago after lunch but Marie spent the afternoon with her.

May 12 – Janet goes to Grant South today. The day started with an early rise, breakfast in the dining hall and a heavy workout all day. She is getting bored where she is and is ready to get on with the new program. Tally Ho!

I was no stranger to leg or knee problems. As a kid and into my twenties, I was a figure skater. Although resultant knee injuries prevented me from heading to national competitions, I skated three to four times a week for a couple hours daily. I also took ballet lessons to work on balance and creative training. When I began training for the big jumps, my coach told me that the critical movement during the takeoff for a jump was to keep my "nose over toes." While this was annoying, as my right leg would give out endlessly, I would repeat and repeat the jump. In the early 1990s, I did have my right knee rebuilt. I am very grateful, because I now rely on my right leg since my left side was completely paralyzed.

So it was that ice-skating all those years ago prepared me to learn how to walk correctly again. I was ready and excited to start physical therapy: it was like training for another ice skating competition. The physical therapist and I called it Boot Camp, and I had no idea how difficult it would be. I told the physical therapist, "Just let me get on the bike, I'll ride for a few hours." However, I couldn't even sit straight up in a chair, because my stomach muscles were so weak. At first, I thought this was funny, but I soon realized I was going to need lots of physical therapy. And physical therapy was more complicated, due to my vision problems: I could see somewhat better in my peripheral vision, but straight ahead was very blurry.

I was limited to a lot of the more aggressive exercises due to my lack of vision. Initially, the physical therapists focused on my balance and strengthening my stomach muscles. I would stand between two balance bars and, goofing around, try to swing on both the bars. This was not what the physical therapists wanted me to do. They wanted me to stand on a rubber disc between those bars. I was to use the bars for support and just stand on the disc. I thought, Boring, boring, boring. The truth is, I was so weak, I could barely handle standing there for a few minutes, so I would pull a trick and say I'm a little thirsty. Then, I could sit down. I was always tired and standing up for two minutes was exhausting. So, I sipped the water slowly. Next, they asked me to put some pegs in a hole in a board on a wall. I thought, this is third grade stuff! I could barely do it, given my vision, but I did it slowly. Standing was killing me and holding my arms up was ridiculously painful. Had I turned 70?

They stopped falling for the water trick. I wanted to start working on the walker. Nope, not until I could see. I was furious! Ok fine, I thought. My eyes aren't getting better, but

I will roll my wheelchair out in the hallway and try to get out of it by myself, pull myself up and use one of the bars on the walls and practice, no one will see me. That didn't work: I was scolded and told I could fall and hurt myself and that if I tried that again I would be tied to my bed. Good grief! So, I cried hysterically. The physical therapist proceeded to work with me, but I was so tired and sad. On occasion, my leg started shaking, a neurological condition called clonus. It would happen to me when my muscles were tired.

The plan was to continue working on strengthening my muscles until I could have my eye surgery. The surgery, called bilateral vitrectomy, is performed when the fluid in the eye is clouded with blood and debris. That fluid, called vitreous, is replaced with a saline solution. The doctors hoped that the blood debris would clear up on its own, and they also waited until I could be weaned off the blood thinners. For these reasons, the surgeries did not occur until July and August. Nevertheless, I made progress in PT with my arm and core muscles, slowly but surely.

May 13 – Janet now can walk several steps with a walker. Today she went to physical therapy in the morning and saw a neurological ophthalmologist in the afternoon. He said that brain aneurysms are usually accompanied with bleeding in the eyes and suggests that Janet see a retinologist. Dr. Hawley, pulmonologist, wants to take out the trachea tube next week. Janet has some fears of falling since her bed is near the window but staff will move it away from the window in the morning; other than that she seems to be in good spirits and her tennis shoes are working out well. She can walk better in them than in the knobby shoes supplied by the hospital.

May 14 – Dr. Ridenour said that Janet's left eye has a clot and this is obstructing her vision to the point that he can't see in either eye and she can't see out. He hopes this will clear and no surgery will be needed.

Also today, Janet had six hours of therapy and was able to walk up stairs with the aid of a walker. At the end of the day she asked what would be the chances of her having another aneurysm and was told that the possibility was there but that chances were very slight.

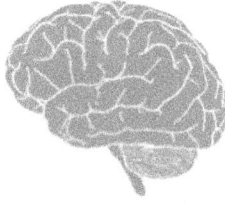

CHAPTER 12

Paris and Nicky

I had finally made it to Grant South. The nurses were so excited to see me go, they cheered, "Give them hell, Janet!" as I left. I was a challenging patient. I had the habit of giving everyone a bath when they would bathe me, and they were ready for me to move on. I was looking forward to new surroundings and a new routine called "boot camp." I remember actually being allowed to wear underwear!! Yes, I graduated to underwear and real clothing. Holy cow, my diva days were coming back!!

I did have a slight shock when my mom bought me a powder blue bra at Kohl's: my breast size had changed because all of the steroids I had been given while in intensive care. Go figure: brain surgery equals bigger boobs. My bra size actually went up to a triple D. I thought, how awful and incomprehensible to manage such large breasts in a powder blue bra! As she helped me try to get my gigantic breasts into the new bra, my nurse said, "Ok, let's get Sally and Suzy in here." She struggled, tugged, and pulled me into that bra. So, my head was partly bald and now my breasts were ridiculously circus-like and huge. I decided they would not be called Sally and Suzy but Paris and Nicky. I wanted to put a spin on my ginormous breasts and make them fabulous! So, I corrected the nurse and said, "Excuse me, they will now be called Paris and Nicky." With lots of laughs, every nurse and staff member who helped me dress became familiar with Paris and Nicky. Onward and upward, to boot camp with Paris and Nicky in the powder blue bra!

Boot camp was aptly named; it felt like some sort of military school. After an early breakfast, it was only work all day long: physical therapy, speech therapy, recreational therapy, and occupational therapy. I wanted to nap in between these sessions, but there was no time: I was supposed to be learning how to tie my shoes and put on my powder blue bra. Social integration was also part of the program: I needed to catch up on current events and eat with the other patients. Since I was blind, I preferred to eat alone; I inevitably knocked over my drink, a huge embarrassment, and I still worried I would choke.

Eventually, I did make the effort to go to the cafeteria – not as much to make friends but because I was hungry! It wasn't always a pleasant experience, however, because it reminded me how disabled I was. Occasionally an old man would throw up at the table, but luckily I was blind and didn't see anything. I just heard the barfing and crying from the old gentlemen who mumbled, "It's hard getting old." I thought, "Where the heck am I? Did they leave me in an old folks' home? This is a place just like where my grandma and grandpa lived. Oh God, my life is over. My Zsa Zsa self is trapped in a nursing home."

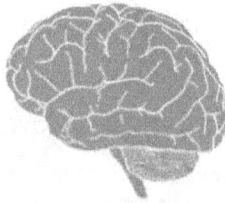

CHAPTER 13

Channeling My Inner Zsa Zsa

At lunch, I would always hear sad stories. Strangely, the other patients seemed to have no idea why they were there; they were just as disoriented as I was. One wheelchair-bound girl kept asking about her horse, but her mom would tell her every day that her horse died since the "accident." From what I could tell, this girl had been thrown from her horse. She cried and cried.

Even though there was a lot of crying going on in that rehab center, it was interspersed with humor. It was odd how the men liked to one-up each other about their motorcycle accidents or bar room brawls, even though they were in wheelchairs. My favorite was an old guy who, from what I could see with my peripheral vision, wore a red flannel shirt and resembled my dad. He was a little goofy. One day, when my friend Katie and her newborn daughter Caroline were visiting me, this old man told us that he had just seen my parents. He said my mom was walking my dad. We were excited thinking we were going to see both of them. That is, until this old nutty guy said, "Your dad is a pig, right? Well your mom had him on a leash and was taking him for a walk." I was so amused! I looked at Katie who pulled Caroline closer to her. I winked at her and after he left, I said, "This place is full of crazies." She tried to explain to me that some of the people were sick and were being treated at the hospital; I really didn't completely understand.

Every day, I heard alarms going off as patients tried to escape from the hospital. One patient kept trying to go to Olive Garden; I guess she didn't like the cafeteria's food. I liked the food, but I still ended up wearing most of my meals; my perpetually fuzzy vision meant my hospital gown was always covered with salad or chocolate mousse. I was a glamorpuss!

By the end of May, my delusions had mostly subsided, but reality became another kind of prison. I was alone in this rehab hospital with older people who could hardly remember what year it was; except for our age difference, I realized that I was just like them. I began to comprehend just how sick I must have been. I now knew that I needed to relearn everything that used to be easy. I had to think about each step. Physical therapy was a frustrating marathon, and there seemed to be no hope of permanently graduating from my wheelchair to a walker or cane because I still couldn't see very well at all.

I finally realized that Bogie was gone. My parents continued to travel back and forth; my brother visited regularly. It was beginning to dawn on me, the disruption I had caused in their lives. I had had a boyfriend at the start of this whole drama but, like a coward, he had disappeared.

Hoping to feel better about everything, I attempted to put on make-up. Maybe looking sassy would help. But since I couldn't see, I ended up wearing eyeliner as lipstick and mascara got all over my face. I was furious! So, I just began wearing my black Gucci sunglasses. Since I was on the blood thinner Coumadin, the nurse would stand by the shower while I shaved so I wouldn't bleed to death, I guess. For heaven's sake, things were out of control: I was hairy like I had been camping in the Grand Canyon for months! The nurse and I both laughed about how I needed some cleaning up.

I would complain to my dad about how long my toenails were and he would take a nail file and file them down; he was very concerned that they weren't straight. I had a pity party one day, crying and asking, "Why me?" and "When will I be my old self again?" My mom sat on my hospital bed and hugged me. She promised to bring in a woman to give me a manicure and haircut.

It seemed to me I had been punished with this brain aneurysm (a medical term I still didn't understand). One of the nurses told me the story of a patient who had been in a wheelchair but promised to come back walking. Well, this patient did and had made a difference in peoples lives. The nurse told me this was my chance to make a difference. I was annoyed at first, but that did get me thinking and eventually asking questions.

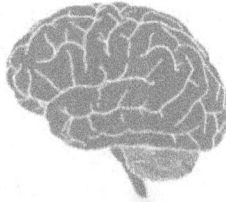

CHAPTER 14

Piecing the Puzzles Together

Nothing got past my Dad when I was in boot camp.

May 15 – Janet is still concerned that she might have another aneurysm. In spite of reassurances by Dr. Shehadi and several other doctors that the odds are very, very slight, it is a thought that she has trouble putting to rest. It is on her mind daily. In spite of this distraction, she has had six therapy sessions of 30-45 minutes each since arriving at Grant South and she has walked increasingly longer distances with the aid of a walker. Her vision is improving and staff say they are very pleased with her progress.

May 16 – Janet has had a quiet day; Katie came by with her baby and they visited. She can see better but is still afraid to be alone since she was alone when the aneurysm burst. Grant South staff plan to have an evaluation next week to set goals to gauge her recovery progress. Janet's goal is to get out and go home. Dr. Hawley wants to do another bronchoscope next week and take out the trachea tube if no longer needed. Janet still expresses concern about whether she could have another aneurysm and has discussed this again with Dr. Shehadi and Dr. Mackessey and staff. It has been said that she may need to have angiograms at yearly or at bi-annual intervals to determine whether any new aneurysms form.

Wanting to know more about brain aneurysms, I followed doctors around the hallway in my wheelchair asking questions. I even went to the medical records department. I suspected something was up due to the lack of information. I was acting like a typical reporter. A psychologist rattled off some stats about brain aneurysms which were no help since I couldn't even balance my checkbook. Remember that math part? But my parents tried to convince me I would not have another brain aneurysm. My family was trying whatever they could to make me feel better.

May 17 – Janet usually eats breakfast and lunch with the group but today, after six sessions of therapy, she had dinner in her room. She walks behind a grocery cart and all her muscles hurt. Vision in the left eye is a tiny bit better and she is beginning to be able to pick out colors of some the foods on her plate such as spinach, rice and macaroni. The cystitis has cleared up; she feels good and today is going to get a manicure, a facial and a haircut.

This was a nice treat, except when I asked how my haircut looked and my mom said I looked like Sinead O'Connor (ya know the bald pop singer), I thought that either my mom didn't know what she was talking about or I had a horrific haircut. What's next? I was kinda hoping I'd resemble Mariah Carey!

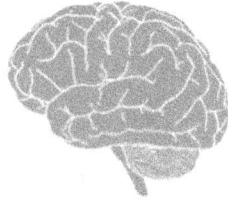

CHAPTER 15

Female Role Models

I still had so many questions until my co-worker Val Turner came to visit me. She sat at my bedside and told me exactly what happened. I am sure my family tried to tell me, but I don't think I was at the point to absorb the information. Val quietly explained about the rupture, my parents flying in from Chicago, how I nearly died, and what a miracle I was. We both cried and cried. It took a lot for someone to sit with me and be so honest and compassionate.

Val and I first met in 2002 when we shared an office at WTVN. I was in a new town and homesick, living for the first time away from Glen Ellyn. I wondered if I made the right decision to move for a job and a new relationship. Val became like a sister to me in that challenging and confusing time. She and I worked on a commission-only basis in a male-dominated environment. A single mom, she was pleasant and polite, a highly intelligent go-getter. She worked in sales with me and gave me lots of insightful tips on how to close a deal. She taught me how to creatively sell sponsorship packages as well as work the computer system. She was a great encouragement to me.

My mom started her life breaking barriers: In 1950-51 the master's political science program at University of Chicago included only two women. One was my mom, Marie Panor Sutherland. The first piece of advice from my mom I listened to was when she told me never shy away from a new adventure in life. She told me to take a chance in life, so I took the job to Ohio and made the move. I hesitated to move away from home, I am not sure why. Her advice stemmed from personal experience. She moved away from her family in Wash D.C. to work over-sees in Germany. Returning to D.C. later with my dad to raise two children, Mom took advantage of the history at our doorstep. She worked for political causes and learned all about American history. We often drove past the Watergate hotel and she told us about the scandal. We would scream Nixon as we drove by and giggled. My parents weren't so amused. My mom watched kids in the neighborhood and sent my brother and me to a desegregated school in Rockville, Maryland. Later when we moved to Chicago, she volunteered for a community shelter for homeless people with drug problems and then for a family counseling service.

After my brain aneurysm, she became my best friend. She is admired by all of my girlfriends. She never gave up on me when I was facing a rough time in the ICU. One of the nurses told her I was a fighter and to not to lose hope. My mom still remembers those kind words. She still reminds me about being a fighter. She battled with me to live, to walk, to re-learn how to drive, to socialize, even to step over the curb and get out of the tub. She mourned with me when Bogie died. She's the embodiment of endless love and support.

My paternal grandmother, Dorothy Susan Ripley Sutherland, who lived past the age of 102, was very proper, classy, and well educated. During the summer she drove the motorboat while my grandfather took his morning ski. She was one of the first women to graduate from the University of Illinois business school. When I worked in radio and would whimper about the low pay and hours, my grandma told me, "Suck it up." I was quite shocked to hear that coming from her mouth. I expected, "Oh poor Janet, life can be rough. We will support you for the rest of your life." Nope. So all the while I was pushing my "nose over toes," learning how to sit up, put my clothes on, and get better (so I could go home, go back to work and move back to Chicago), I was hearing Grandma in my head: "Suck it up."

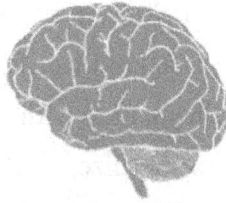

CHAPTER 16

A Dream

I was loaded with concerns: is God mad at me, will I adjust to my new life, and how will I function alone? I was full of anxiety then, and I still experience it now. I am learning that anxiety comes with being a brain aneurysm survivor. Also, being forgetful is common. In my case, I wouldn't remember things and would get upset because I was used to being a snappy, fast-talking, five-steps-ahead-of-the-subject type of person. In the months directly after my rupture, I was just struggling to figure out what day and time it was! I wanted to bust out of this slow moving, confused shell and get back to my former Zsa Zsa reporter-self!

My dad described more frustrations I faced:

May 18 - The blood clot in the left eye is beginning to dissolve but a lot more of it needs to dissolve before her vision is normal. Speech went well but the therapist is trying to slow her down so she does not speak so rapidly. She has a tendency to slough off new topics; she is alert about her therapy but is still anxious about the future. There is the possibility of another aneurysm and she has the difficult task of relearning old skills that are ever so hard to relearn. She now remembers a dream she had about Jeanine Mahon, deacon at St. Mark's Church in Glen Ellyn, IL, when she was in her coma. In it, Janet saw a bright light and told Jeanine that she was afraid. Jeanine told her not to be afraid. Penny (Janet's cousin) called near the end of the afternoon; they had a good conversation and Janet felt reassured she would recover.

It was hard to figure out if the dream was a visit from a guardian angel, which I tend to believe. Jeanine was my friend from church who gave me spiritual guidance when I was in high school. I remember, as I was fighting for life during my brain aneurysm, seeing a light and kicking and screaming and saying, "I am not going to go. No way!" Realizing that the impending death experience was real has given me a new perspective on people, life experiences, God, and making a difference in this world.

May 19 – I talked to Janet on the phone after returning to Glen Ellyn; she is understandably concerned about the future, in view of her present difficulty in seeing and in using her left arm and leg. Within a week, she plans to set up an appointment with Dr. Epstein. The hospital is talking about a mid-June date for her to go home in which case she would continue therapy at an outpatient clinic in Arlington. At present she is in therapy from 8:00am to 3:00pm and making good progress. She can walk with the aid of a walker and has made a few steps on her own, unaided. She is being very brave, moving ahead in spite of her fears; her dreams about Jeanine have comforted her and she says she had a dream of me sitting by her bed telling her everything would be OK, perhaps recalling the afternoons, during her coma, when I did just that. These dreams are helping her fend off anxieties about the unknown ahead.

May 20 - Hallucinations seem to be gone and her case manager says she will be going home in mid-June, probably around June 14. Janet is still concerned about another aneurysm and has many fears and tears about that and her vision handicap. She can't focus the right eye and both eyes have blood in them from burst blood vessels due to the aneurysm. However, vision is improving slowly in the left eye and she begins to see colors. I think it would be good for her to have another talk with Dr. Shehadi about these fears to understand that although no absolute certainty can be given to reassure her, the chances are extremely slight that a burst aneurysm will recur. She is still working hard in therapy-making more progress in walking with the aid of a walker and in being able to raise her left arm.

The psychologist has recommended Zoloft for anxieties but it makes Janet sleepy during therapy sessions. I think we need to keep reassuring her that everything will work out and that she will make a full recovery. This will not be easy and will only come one step, one day at a time.

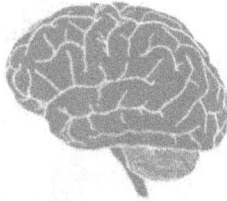

CHAPTER 17

The Brace- Not Christian Louboutin's

May 21 – Janet has been fitted with a lightweight, four-inch plastic Velcro brace, because her left ankle collapses when she puts weight on it. The brace is intended not only to strengthen the ankle but also to help keep her from becoming exhausted after long physical therapy sessions. Related to another matter, Dr. Rindler seems to have some hesitation about releasing Janet for home while she still needs a walker. The walker would make it difficult for her to get in and out of bathrooms and go up and down stairs. It is also important for her morale that she be able to function independently.

The brace, which medical professionals call an ankle-foot orthosis, or AFO, was the first of about a dozen that were created for me. It sported a picture of Donald Duck; apparently I was now five years old. Yes, I had lost my sense of humor. "Please get me something cute, but not kindergarten-cute," was what I was thinking because the brace would not fit in my shoes - unless I planned on wearing stark white orthopedic shoes for the rest of my life. Which I did not.

Technology has improved such that my current brace does not impact the shoes I wear. It wraps around my lower left leg, stopping under my knee, and it is very small compared to the Donald Duck brace. I wear it not for strengthening my ankle but because of nerve damage: I cannot feel my left foot. An electronic pulse shocks a muscle in my leg causing my left foot to go up and down, so I can walk. It was not covered by my insurance, and it cost $5000. It works, and I can wear normal shoes, but it does look like a home monitoring device, so some people joke with me that I am a crook. Hey I'd rather look like a felon and be fashionable and comfortable. Yes, it's that important!

At this point, I was mostly still in a wheelchair; I used the Donald Duck brace when practicing with my walker.

May 25 – With her walker and brace, Janet walked 150 feet in one stretch. The psychiatrist came to visit; he remarked about the progress she is making. Many friends called and stopped by to visit. Janet's spirits were lifted but she still has problems recognizing people and seeing the hands on the wall clock in her room. Although walking has improved, her ankle still needs to be wrapped because the nerves were damaged when the aneurysm burst. Friday 5/31 she has an appointment with the neurologist and on Wednesday 6/1, an appointment with Dr. Epstein.

May 26 – Dr. Ahee came by to visit and said recent tests showed that the clots in the left leg as well as the lungs have dissolved; they are gone. This is great news! The damage that could have resulted if they had not dissolved had been a big worry for weeks. Other good news: today Janet was able to see a little bit better and her ankle seems to be getting stronger.

I'd been told that the clots in my leg were gone. The doctor was so excited, but I started to cry. I had forgotten that I had clots in my lungs and legs. What a mess I had been. The doctor must have left my room feeling a little defeated, since I had greeted his news with tears. Now I was thinking, okay, great, one less thing to worry about, but what else is going on with me? I guess I am a little bit of a pessimist. But can you blame me? My memory was terrible.

May 27 & 28 – Janet walked for an hour with the aid of a hand-held pole and did well playing a memory game. She was also able to give herself a sponge bath with her injured left hand, but she still has difficulty seeing the food on her plate. Staff give her the food and then leave; she has to figure out where it is and learn how to eat without help. This is a drill to develop coping mechanisms.

After lunch she walked down the corridor holding on to a bar and went for speech lessons which were easy. Talking has always has been natural for Janet and her speech was not affected by the aneurysm, it was only inhibited by the trache.

The brain aneurysm affected so many parts of my body: my eyes, legs, arms, and even my bladder. The rehab center limited the amount of times I could use the bathroom. I was told if I used the bathroom more than once on my own, I would be tied to the bed. Pure hell, but I now understand why. My brain needed to be trained that I didn't always have to go to the bathroom. It seems like every habit, every movement had to be retrained in my brain. This is why I was always tired.

My therapists blamed my poor handwriting and rapid speech on the brain injury. They didn't know that those characteristics are part of me. This made some of my therapy sessions more laborious. My family and friends had to continually tell the therapists that they were fighting a losing battle; my penmanship was not going to improve nor my speech slow down.

May 29 & 31 - A couple friends visited, and Janet had speech and physical therapy for two hours. Her eyesight has improved slightly. On Sunday 5/31 she went to a picnic in the cafeteria and walked with the walker to a nearby park. Aides restrict her from going to the restroom more than once every two hours to redevelop urinary control after wearing a catheter for so many weeks. She is taking medication to fight yeast infections as well as an antibiotic.

June 1 - Janet has been in Grant South for 20 days. Soon she will be able to have the stomach tube removed (these were for additional nutrient intake) and will be able to go home where she will continue therapy twice a week. For two weeks she has had headaches. Dr. Mallick says these are caused by her scalp stretching as healing from the craniotomy continues. Janet is worried that the clamp at the incision is getting loose, but Dr. Mackessey says it can't come loose and not to worry.

Janet walked the stairs and the length of the hall and back; her posture was very good, a big improvement over several weeks ago. She had three sessions of physical and occupational therapy as well as speech therapy. She will be on Coumadin for six months. She is on a total of 16 different medications but some will soon be dropped off.

My dad was able to capture in his journal the nose over toes technique I used from my figure skating days. My ice skating coach Barbara Davis would teach us to skate just like the physical therapist was teaching me how to get up from a chair: I would push myself up off the chair leaning forward with my nose over my toes.

June 2 – Janet met with Dr. Epstein and he said that she has Terson syndrome. This means that blood for some reason travels from the brain to the eyeball, probably down the optic nerve, and the blood causes cloudy vision which takes time to work out before vision is clear again. Surgery is an option but only if it does not clear up naturally. This can take a long time in a young person because the vitreous humor is dense.

In an older person, vitreous is less dense and the blood clears out sooner. Janet will see Dr. Ridenour on Friday at 10:30 am to hear his assessment of the situation. Janet feels she has made great strides, which she has, and she wants to go home on June 11. However, one problem is that she needs help in supporting 50 percent of her weight when she takes steps and when transferring to the toilet. The risk of a fall in the bathroom seems small, but when going up stairs the risk seems great. We asked staff to go to bat for her with the insurance company, requesting that she be permitted to stay in Grant South until she can support 75 percent of her weight as therapists recommend. This would cut down on the risks of falling. Her physical therapist, Julie, says that progress in walking is gradual but steady; Janet's vision is a big problem and handicaps her when shifting weight as she walks. Another railing on the stairs to the second floor of her apartment is needed (so she can better support herself when going up and down stairs).

June 2-6 – Janet had two sessions of occupational therapy, one of physical therapy and one of speech therapy. On the 2nd she walked without a walker. The same regimen took place on the 4th and she also stepped up on a box with her right foot. On the 5th she walked up and down the stairs using her right foot only and on *the 6thshe was told that she would be going home on the 11that which time she hopes to be walking without a walker. On the 6th she also went for a stroll in the park next to the medical center using a walker and hopes to return to the park on Friday.*

June 7 - Marie and I attended physical therapy and got hands-on instruction on how to help Janet transfer from chair to bed. Marcia Gill explained how to help Janet get up on a bed by keeping her left leg bent so she can push up and then blocking her left foot to keep it from sliding when she transfers from a bed to wheelchair. She also learned a pick-up exercise by stretching to the side to give an object to someone and then, after getting in a wheelchair, to reach back to the left to get the lock and swing the arm in place. Marcia said Janet would receive counseling and other outpatient services as needed. The philosophy is that three days of exercise is enough since she needs to recover in between sessions.

The rehab hospital was preparing many of us to go into the outside world. I wasn't ready to be labeled "handicapped." My dad discussed some of our activities but I didn't tell anyone how embarrassed I was to be considered "disabled," riding in a "disabled" bus and using a wheelchair. Yep, I was more concerned about how I looked than anything else. I had never been out in public in a wheelchair. Oh my God!! This is my worst nightmare: I was half bald, no makeup, weird clothes, I couldn't even see my outfit to pick it out and I just was not myself. It felt like I had lost complete control as to who I was and what I looked like.

June 8 & 9 - A staff person arrived with applications for handicap stickers. Janet went on an outing to a department store to buy greeting cards, lip balm and other things. Vision in her left eye is improving somewhat, as she is able to see shadows in the center of the eye. The right eye is not improving as well.

Dr. Redd came by and introduced herself; Janet liked her very much. Dr. Mackessey also dropped in and explained that Janet's headaches are caused by sinus infections. One item of good news was that her baldness, caused from lying on her back with her head on the pillow for three weeks when in a coma, is going away; her hair is beginning to grow back now that she is able to get around.

Not having much hair is a HUGE issue for women but I guess my dad didn't realize how I was almost traumatized by it. At this point, things were getting more real, handicap stickers and baldness, and I was glad now, in a way, to be blind to that hot mess! Furthermore, they gave me a donut-shaped pillow to sleep on. My humiliation level was nearing 10... and you wonder why I needed the anxiety meds! I had no hair and I was sleeping on a pillow with a hole in it! Upon introducing the new Styrofoam pillow, the nurse explained that it was for the bald spot on the back of my head. I put it on, looking ridiculous. The nurse crossed his arms as he stood there looking at me; he seemed super pleased with himself. He smirked and said, "It fits."

According to my Dad's journal, the process of being discharged from the hospital involved many sessions, none of which I remember except for headaches.

On June 9, we had more training in how to assist Janet in transferring from one location to another. Dr. Mackessey made arrangements for a CAT scan to determine any additional cause of her headaches. He expects that the jaw line and muscle cuts made during surgery as well as bone growth during the healing process are the culprits. Also today Janet had three sessions of physical therapy, two sessions of on the job training, and one session of speech therapy.

Since my experience, I have met many brain aneurysm survivors who have shunts in their heads, but I don't have one. A shunt is tubing that drains cerebral fluid from a condition called hydrocephalus. My dad's journal indicates that the doctors suspected I may have suffered from hydrocephalus, but they ruled it out.

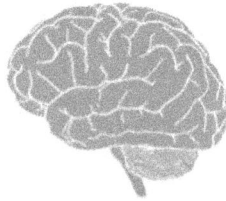

CHAPTER 18

Another Aneurysm

At the time of my emergency brain surgery in March, Dr. Ronald Budzik had identified a second aneurysm. The decision was made to wait and treat it after the ruptured aneurysm was under control. According to my dad's journal,

Several questions have come up regarding continuing issues: whether the fluid pressure build-up on the brain could possibly cause a stroke and whether the 4 mm aneurysm on the left side of the brain may need to be coiled. The increased size of the ventricles in the brain is also a concern and seems to have been caused by the build-up of fluid pressure. It was decided Janet should have a CAT scan in one week and follow up with Dr. Joseph Shehadi on June 24. Her right eyebrow has yet to respond to muscle control following the craniotomy; also, she has been on Coumadin for two months and will be on it for two more months before this clot reduction therapy is completed.

My second brain aneurysm was coiled in August. A coil is like a slinky that is inserted into the aneurysm. So, we all could breathe a sigh of relief.

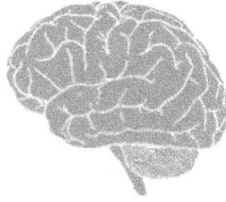

CHAPTER 19

Going Home

June 12 – Great News! Janet goes home. Her great friend Katie has put up Welcome Home signs on the road to her apartment unit with 20 flamingos saying hello. All of us had smiles and cheers. We went for a walk in the evening, pushing Janet in her wheelchair. Although her vision is still extremely limited, causing difficulty when she walks, she can see to put on her mascara.

My dad and the neighbor next door managed to get a ramp to my door and lifted my wheelchair into my apartment. I was home! The phone calls began right away: first, it was my best friend Becky from Illinois. At the sound of her voice, I started crying. I tried to explain that yes, I'm home but I'm also blind and paralyzed. She reassured me and promised her love and prayers. Next, the former minister from our church in Glen Ellyn, Father Cole, called to welcome me home and we talked briefly. I felt so glad to hear from him: he reassured me about my experience of seeing Jeanine in my dreams.

The excitement was exhilarating and exhausting. I tried to transfer myself from the wheelchair to the sofa as my dad talked to more friends on the phone, but I fell face first into the pillows. I thought Oh well, something to work on tomorrow. I reached my dad and leaned on him as he chatted gleefully, spreading the good news.

My happiness was tempered by one thing: Bogie was not there waiting for me. The urn containing his ashes was there instead. I burst into hysterical tears, and my parents cried too. We were overwhelmed suddenly by all the sad things that had happened in such a short period of time. Questions came flooding back to my mind: Am I going to be wheelchair-bound for the rest of my life? Will I have to go to a blind school or a nursing home? Will I always be a burden to my family?

In the cool of that first evening, my dad took me for a walk in my wheelchair. Reflecting on all of the well-wishers and my parents' loving nearness, I realized that I was blessed despite my condition. My dad kept telling me how heartbroken people would feel if I were not around. That truth had never even occurred to me, but the outpouring of affection I had experienced that day proved it. I sat upright in the wheelchair and thought, Wait a minute! I am not done yet. There are still things I want to do; my life isn't over. Plus, my will isn't written yet. I'm not prepared to die. These people have no idea what kind of funeral I want and I need to write my books and do many, many more things in this world. No, dying was not an option! From that point on I was anxious to get the aneurysm fixed and my vision resolved.

My first night's sleep back in my own bed felt like it lasted for days; it was good to be home.

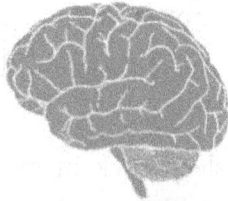

CHAPTER 20

Adjustments

My parents promised to help me until my condition improved enough that I could live on my own. They made huge sacrifices. Mom ended up living with me for 18 months away from my father. She set up appointments with therapists, including psychotherapy to help me adjust to living with a disability. She helped me get around the kitchen and manage the household. She was with me as I learned how to drive again, which wasn't very difficult; in fact, my mom declared, "I'm bored," and we laughed. It wasn't as exhilarating as the first time around, when I was a 16 year old.

My two-story apartment was converted to a one-floor bedroom. My parents started their own physical therapy program for me. At each meal they would insist I use my left hand. I was also required to unload the dryer with my left arm. At night my dad worked on exercises with my arms and legs. He was a drill sergeant, but it all helped.

We had fun living together, although it was like a re-run from my childhood, when my mom always gave us carrot sticks. I began calling home with her "carrotstickland" because every meal involved carrot sticks.

In those first weeks at home, we were all so anxious for my vision to return to normal. Dr. Ridenour had told us that my vision may return slowly, and it was, but we were impatient. My hearing had certainly been vastly accentuated. I could hear the phone begin to ring before anyone else. My sense of smell was also very keen. But there in my Ohio parking lot, when my dad asked if I could read the license plate, I yelled "Yes, it's an Ohio plate!" because I didn't want him to be disappointed.

I was struggling in church, due to the anger I was suppressing against God. In many ways, this felt like the lowest point in my life. I was home which was great. But at dinner with my family but I still embarrassed myself, putting my hand in my mom's soup and spilling my own drink. Sometimes I would just sit in my wheelchair, which I still used for long periods of time, listening to inspirational music on my Walkman and saying the Lord's Prayer over and over in my head, hoping God would hear me. I couldn't believe that God didn't protect me from this brain aneurysm and the destruction it had caused to my entire life and my family's life.

I spoke with an Episcopal minister who helped me when he said it's OK to be mad at God. He told me that God would help me deal with the results of the aneurysm, and He did. I am writing a book, raising funds, and creating support groups. But during those early days, when life was trying to find a new normal, my emotions and thoughts bounced from one extreme to the other. Here is what my dad recorded of my second full day home:

June 13 - Janet and I went to church; she had been on the prayer list for two months. It was good to get out and everyone was happy to see her. Her spirits were high and we went for a walk in the evening.

June 14 - Janet went to outpatient therapy. She had an evaluation and staff were impressed by the movement of her left arm and leg. She has made much improvement as indicated by the 20 lb. squeeze in her left hand. She is able to stand up normally with good balance and posture. She will not take steps unassisted until the physical therapist approves her doing so which we expect will be on Tuesday. Janet saw herself in the mirror and was able to see her hair, eyebrows, and face. She was also able to see outlines but not full views down to her waist. Dr. Ridenauer guessed that there was more improvement in her peripheral vision than in the center of her eye since she was not able to see the big "E" on the center of the eye chart.

What my dad omitted in his journal was that seeing myself for the first time was heartbreaking. I looked so different, and I was in a wheelchair!!! Oh my God! I would cry and cry. My parents were just happy I was alive. I *was* happy to be alive, but I wasn't the real me. On top of everything else, the guy I was dating had fallen off the face of the earth, and I felt rejected.

My brother Mark drove six hours from his home to Ohio just to take me out to the movies. I used my cane, but Mark held my left hand as we walked into the theater. Although I am older, he always acted like my big brother when we were kids: he watched out for me. Having Mark by my side that day was a comforting reminder of our childhood. I remember once when I was little, I packed a suitcase and planned to run away from home and my brother cried for me to come back. Now here he was, helping steer me over the curbs and past all those strangers' faces. It was great to have him there with me.

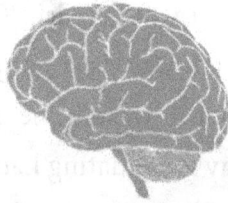

CHAPTER 21

Nose Over Toes

June 15 - The physical therapist, Jaya, urged Janet to work her left leg and not baby it. Jaya would say, "Sit down and stand up on your own without help. Push yourself to the limit point of being able to do the exercise correctly but don't go beyond that point and develop bad habits."

Jaya was pleasant and upbeat. After introducing herself and doing her initial evaluation, she beamed out to us, "OK, Miss Janet, we are gonna get you out of this wheelchair!" I thought Really?! My parents couldn't believe it. At this point, I did use a walker but only around the house: from the car to the front door, or to get to the bathroom. Otherwise, I still used a wheelchair for most movement. We made a bunch of appointments and started a round of outpatient physical therapy sessions.

Meeting Miss Jaya was just what we needed. All three of us were tired; emotionally, we had lost hope. My parents needed someone to tell them that I would get better. Lugging my wheelchair in and out of vehicles while they tried to get around Columbus was also tiring for my parents. Jaya was very positive and supportive and she gave us lots of details about my therapy. She even gave my parents tips for navigating the Columbus roads. My dad wanted to know what he could do to help me; he took careful notes during the sessions with Jaya and did the exercises at home with me.

Use of my left hand came back quickly, but what I wanted most was to be out of my wheelchair. Jaya wanted me to set goals, so I told her I needed to be walking with my walker for a Fourth of July party. Doctors did not want me to exclusively use a walker until my eyesight had returned, but I was still pushing for July 3. As a motivation, the General Manager got us tickets to a big fireworks show. He was a great supporter as I began to heal. Someone had anonymously paid for Bogie's vet bill, and it may have been him. As it turned out, I skipped the big fireworks show but did attend a smaller party using a walker, my parents by my side.

June 16 - Janet did exercises and was able to put more weight on her left foot in order to hold it flat on the ground. We went to a party at Clear Channel, the radio station where Janet worked, and were welcomed by all; there were lots of tears when people saw Janet. They went to great lengths to make her feel comfortable; her desk was all fixed up and she was able to visit old friends. Marie and I were made to feel at home and given a grand welcome. It was a great afternoon.

June 17 - Janet went to therapy and made good progress keeping her foot on the ground but it was hard, requiring her to keep the knee slightly flexed and not locked. She also did push-ups against a bar and can be doing them at home against a wall. She also worked on mini-deep knee bends. She was given an organizational test and scored in the 95th percentile.

June 18 - She had a CAT scan to check on the clip and other things, e.g., ventricles and fluid pressure. The scan was completed as scheduled but the conference with Dr. Shehadi had to be rescheduled until 11:00 on Tuesday; however, we were able to pick up her walker.

June 20 – Janet and I went to church while Marie stayed home. Janet was able to see out of the corners of her eyes but her primary vision in center field and most of the peripheral areas are still gone. Her hearing was keener than normal, compensating for her lack of sight. In the afternoon Janet and Marie went to the garden store and bought plants and mulch. Janet camped under an umbrella on the porch. She now is able to transfer from *wheelchair to car to bathroom without someone spotting where to place her feet.*

Freedom in the bathroom is something I took for granted, before the aneurysm. I never thought to enjoy sitting on the toilet, alone, for as long as I wanted. Now I could do that. Also, I found that wearing underwear is exciting without a catheter. It was like Christmas at my apartment!! Never mind that I had a trache hole in my neck and lots of scars. These things all reminded me how lucky I was to be alive. My diminished eyesight, however, was a continual frustration. I still had not been able to investigate brain aneurysms online to satisfy my curiosity.

In July 2004, I had a vitrectomy in my left eye, a procedure that removed the blood and debris from behind my eye. I was awake during the procedure at Grant Medical Center and could hear Dr. Ridenour talking to his operating room staff; they commented about the amount of blood that he found. Dr. Ridenour's instrument broke during the procedure but he was able to remove everything needed. He was excited about the success of the procedure and gave my parents a thumbs-up as they wheeled me into recovery. We were told not to expect any results soon. I had the same surgery in my right eye in August.

Although the eye surgery went well, post-op care was a little more complicated than we expected. It involved the application of eye drops throughout the day and night, and this interrupted daily functions and sleep patterns. Another key to recovery was making sure the water bubble that the surgeon had placed on the macula in my eye didn't move. To this end, I could only sleep on my side; my parents had to wake up and check on me in the night, rolling me back to my side if I moved. The air bubble was keeping my macula flat so it didn't wrinkle while it healed.

For six weeks after each surgery, I spent multiple hours each day staring at the floor with my head pressed on a table. To pass the time, I listened to the TV or books on CD. One time I went to a pool party at a friend's house, determined not to miss the fun times. I sat with my head on the table looking at the floor.

Mom and Dad kept a chart on the wall to monitor the medications and eye drops I needed: names, times, and amounts. My dad, who went back to work part time in Glen Ellyn, set up an office in my upstairs bedroom where he handled all of my insurance bills. He drove back to me and mom in Ohio every few weeks. Those were long days of therapy and eye drops, pills and exercises, looking at the floor and waiting. I was doing my best to keep my nose over toes, encouraged by my parents and Jaya, family and friends.

Almost one year after the bilateral vitrectomy, I had the fierce desire one day to be done with my walker. My body had to re-learn what to do: the pattern in my brain had to be reset. So my dad walked outside with me, around the parking lot and adjoining pond. We walked and walked, because we knew we had to lay down the brain pattern. We walked inside and we walked outside: we walked everywhere we could think of, until four o'clock in the morning. Dad said we're going to lay the brain pattern down. He was as determined as I was.

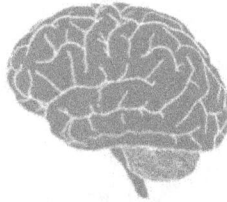

CHAPTER 22

Fun With Mom

My friend Katie and I were big troublemakers before my brain aneurysm; we were thick as thieves. She introduced me to a group of girls and we became, according to my mom, "the Brunch Bunch." I called us the Zsa Zsas. One gal was sweet as can be, but she was never on time. When she showed up for brunch, this gorgeous blonde was always holding a Diet Pepsi with a ring of hot pink lipstick around the can. Katie is a sensible gal who smiles pleasantly and always seems to be able to justify silly behavior. She has the best one-liners (and has always been able to get me to do stupid things.) On one occasion, during my blindness, we were at the mall. Katie convinced me that I could use being blind as an excuse for grabbing the waiter's butt. She dared me and I of course did. I said, "Whoops, I'm sorry sir, I was reaching for my napkin." She thought that was awesome. We laughed and laughed. I asked her why she had me do it, and she said she missed my laugh. It was true: for a long time after my brain aneurysm, I hardly laughed.

Despite all the medications, therapy sessions, and slower walking, I loved being back with the Zsa Zsas. Mom was right there with me. Once, at a birthday celebration, it was obvious that my girlfriends were "on the prowl." My mom exclaimed, "This is fun! These girls are drinking a lot and looking for men." I said Yep, they are. Our table was filled with glammed up, high-maintenance ladies who probably had taken three hours to get ready for the evening. At one point, someone managed to pick up a guy, and he had joined us for dinner. My mom looked around the table and asked me who that man was. I said, "Who knows?" and she laughed, "Someone already picked up a guy!" I said "Ugh, yeah."

I hated to use my walker, because it was So Not Glamorous. One of the girls walked me to the bathroom so I could "fix my face," and when I returned, the whole table was laughing. I wasn't sure why. My mom said, "You lost one of your shoes, but Katie recovered it." Dear God, there I was, struggling to walk through the restaurant thinking I was sassy with the walker, but I was wearing only one shoe. You see, I couldn't feel my left foot. Darn! I am a social outcast! Well at least my mom was enjoying herself.

In 2005, after having surgery on both my eyes and dealing with 12 weeks of staring at the floor, I was ready for some fun. Mark, Dad, and I conspired to coordinate a surprise party for my mom's 75th birthday on November 1; it would be in Chicago. While my brother arranged for a fancy suite at the Sheraton, Mom thought I was planning a small dinner with my friends in the city. She was just looking forward to seeing my dad at their home in Glen Ellyn.

The visit to Chicago typified my post-burst brain aneurysm life: it was thrilling and it was extremely trying. I went to the venue my brother had rented: the penthouse suite was crazy fancy, but I wasn't prepared for the difficulty of using the walker without my mom. I couldn't even walk to the window to see the amazing view of the lake and the Chicago River and all of the skyscrapers lit up because my walker couldn't get around the coffee tables and sofas. Thankfully, my friend Val picked up on my challenge, and she patiently helped me. It wasn't yet on my radar to think about handicapped accessibility, which this place definitely was not.

I was determined and excited to shop at Marshall Field's. However, while navigating the escalators and elevators, it became clear that most shoppers don't have patience for people with walkers. I realized again that things had changed for me. No more trotting down Michigan Avenue. My out-of-town friends, panicked by the Chicago traffic, needed directions, and I couldn't help: my memory was shot. I thought, Wow, you really can't go home anymore. I was so sad, I wanted to cry.

But the surprise was wonderful, for my mom and for me. Although it was my mom's party, everyone applauded when I walked through the door. My friends from Glen Ellyn were crying and my mom's friends were crying. Many people showed up whom I didn't expect, but I think that happens when you dodge death. I told a lot of stories that evening.

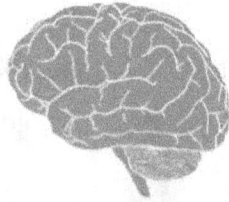

CHAPTER 23

Getting My (New) Groove Back

Being a former radio ad sales rep, I was used to watching the clock. During my blindness, I wore a watch that told me the time audibly. I also still wore a regular watch. One day, after my second vitrectomy, while running an errand with my parents, I looked at my watch and asked, "Is it really two o'clock?" Mom and Dad looked at each other and yelled, "Yes it is, oh my God you can see!!" We were all ecstatic. As soon as I got home, I crawled up the stairs and sent out an email to everyone saying, "Hello all, it's Zsa Zsa!!" People were shocked to receive it, my first email in four months.

A few days later I read the book *The Nannie Diaries*. I had been hearing it was a great book. And I was still all about being on top of the latest trends.

The next thing I did was look online for the Brain Aneurysm Foundation and request info about brain aneurysms. I eventually made contact with the BAF. I realized that its support and educational materials, coupled with an awareness campaign for survivors and caregivers, would help others recover.

I never expected to be taking a driving test when I was 38 years old. There turned out to be so much of life I had to do over! But I wanted my full freedom, and I couldn't return to work before I was driving, so once my vision returned I spent a lot of time practicing in my apartment's parking lot. Within 45 seconds, my mom exclaimed, "I'm bored! You are fine!" I begged her to stay in the car longer because I wanted to ace it and be done with all the silly tests. When my dad came for a visit, he allowed me to drive on a street; he also approved my driving.

On the day of the driving test it was pouring rain. I was using a vehicle that was designed for a paraplegic: a hand shift stopped it, but there were also pedals on the floor like a regular car. So here I was, driving on a country road with two lanes through the pouring rain. In the fields around me I saw the silhouettes of foggy cows. Huge semi-tractor trailers were riding my tail, and the driving conditions were terrible. I could hear my grandma saying, "Suck it up," so I kept going, white knuckles and all. I passed the test!

On our way home after the test, I decided to vote in the Presidential election. The "Vote Here" sign was written in magic marker on poster board, and the letters were running down the paper. I waited in the wrong line for two hours; the polling station was very chaotic. My mom finally got a chair for me. Just as it was my turn to enter the voting cubicle, the machine in it broke, so a 90-year-old election judge voted for me. To this day I am not sure if I voted for the person I wanted to vote for.

Unfortunately, I went back to work too soon. I did this because my boss kept asking me if I were returning to work. He would even ask my co-workers if I was coming back. One of them said, "She's still blind, Jeff." This questioning made my parents nervous that I would lose my health insurance. I had forgotten all about COBRA.

Things had changed, of course: our computer system was different, and I had to relearn how we did business in radio ad sales. My boss privately told my mom that my co-workers had commented, "I wasn't all that there." #MeToo. My mom repeated that to me. Between rumors of my boyfriend cheating on me while I was in the hospital and me "not being all there," I was on the edge.

The General Manager at the radio station made sure there was a handicapped parking space for me. My immediate boss gave me grief and would say to me, "Wow, you really think you are handicapped?" Walking with the brace hurt and was exhausting. Even now, I still get fatigued. I am guarded to go into specifics about my personal challenges due to those kinds of comments.

All of this weird stress and pressure to meet my sales goals caused me to get in my car daily and cold call. I pulled over one day, feeling sick. I drove back to the radio station and spoke to one of my friends who noticed part of my face was drooping. I attempted to drive to the hospital but got lost. One of my friends called and tried to get me to pull over and call 911. I drove back to work. A co-worker called 911 and I was taken to Riverside Hospital. Doctors suspected possibly a TIA, an early sign of a stroke. This was never diagnosed but it was one of the factors in my decision, in September 2006, to move back home to Glen Ellyn. But first, my new purpose in life began to emerge.

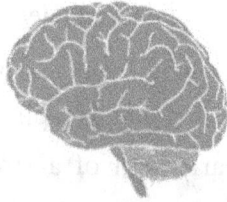

CHAPTER 24

Not Alone

In 2005, I volunteered at Riverside Hospital in the interventional radiology department. I still had cataracts and could barely see. I learned that the ER director, Dr. Bob Walsh, was also a brain aneurysm survivor; my mom read his story to me in the local newspaper. In fact, he had been featured on TLC's *Untold Stories of the ER*, and he had only recently returned to work part-time. I imagined that, with his medical background, he somehow would have had an easier time than I did. In any event, I thought it would be super cool and interesting for both of us to meet.

Though I no longer used a walker, my limp was profound as a friend walked me to Bob's office. I was nervous; I had never met another brain aneurysm survivor, and this man had an impressive job. Bob says he remembers being "awestruck" meeting me because *I* was the first brain aneurysm survivor *he* had ever met. We visited briefly and I bombarded him with ideas like a walk, support group and maybe awareness legislation. I invited Bob to a support group meeting. From the beginning, our common misfortune became our common goal.

Bob and I created a walk to raise $15,000 for The Brain Aneurysm Foundation and a support group for brain aneurysm survivors at The Ohio State University Hospital. We made a great team testifying in front of the Health, Human Services, & Aging committee. We collaborated on brain aneurysm legislation in Ohio: we drafted a law to make September Brain Aneurysm Awareness Month in Ohio.

On May 10 2007 the Ohio General Assembly passed as bill to designate the month of September as "Brain Aneurysm Awareness Month" in Ohio. The published intent of the bill is as follows: The members of the 127th General Assembly feel that it is vitally important that the State of Ohio designate September as Brain Aneurysm Awareness Month. According to the Brain Aneurysm Foundation, brain aneurysms afflict approximately two per cent of Americans, most commonly those aged thirty-five to sixty years. The State encourages and commends private efforts, including those of The Brain Aneurysm Foundation, to enhance funding for aneurysm research, provide educational materials and programs, and create a support network for patients, survivors, and their families.

In remembering the first time we met, Bob says, "I was still a mess." Watching me limp out of his office that day, he welled up with emotion; it was relief in knowing "I was not the only one (to have survived a brain aneurysm). I came to a sudden realization (that) I was not alone."

This is very important for survivors to know. Bob said that first year of his recovery was a mixture of happiness to be alive and the almost "overwhelming realization of what had happened, how come I survived, how come I didn't have any deficits and (how it ended up as) a positive emotional experience."

Bob has a son, three grandchildren, and a daughter who works at OSU. His wife Betsy is retired, and Bob is teaching online at Franklin University Healthcare Management. According to Bob, "Life is good".

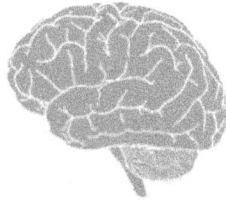

CHAPTER 25

Secret Sauce

I am embarrassed to admit that my ruptured brain aneurysm in 2004 was so severe that it caused massive brain damage. I am not going to sugarcoat it. Dr. Amin Hanjani, the neurosurgeon who took over my case when I moved back to Chicago, reviewed my new scans and said, "Here is the damage." I said, "Damage?" She said, "Yes, brain damage." I thought Whoa, I am super fabulous! What is she talking about?! I put on my typical game face and listened to her review of my CAT scans. Of course, brain aneurysm ruptures and outcomes affect everyone differently, but in this book I offer some tips based on my experience. I developed some weird phobias transitioning from the walker to the cane and in transitioning from the hospital back into regular life.

First, I would freak out whenever I heard ambulance sirens and helicopters. Second, it was tough to go to a movie using my cane and not my walker. I was convinced I was going to tip over because I had nothing to hold onto. Also, stepping up onto a curb without holding onto anything scared me because there were no railings to hold onto. Driving on the expressway was horrifying. A neuropsychologist told me during a session, "You don't want to freeze up on the expressway while passing a semi truck and get in an accident and back in a wheelchair, do you?" After that, I could barely drive on the highway for thinking I was going to end up smashing into a semi. What was that doctor thinking, saying that to a patient?! At that point, I still couldn't remember the date, but I could remember unfortunate comments from a doctor. Things like that could be paralyzing.

Another challenging issue was crowds, because too much noise caused me lots of anxiety. After my list grew to ten issues, I sought out counseling. My psychologist suggested we use a technique for post-traumatic syndrome disorder called EMDR. EMDR (I nicknamed it Secret Sauce) stands for Eye Movement Desensitization and Reprocessing and is a psychotherapy treatment. Because of my eye surgeries, my therapist used hand-tapping and audio stimulation (rather than directing lateral eye movements) to redirecting negative thoughts or disturbing life experiences. So basically, anytime I would hear an ambulance I would tap my leg and train myself to think, "Someone is getting help." And, before taking a step over a curb, I learned to tap my leg and think to myself, "Nose over toes." This eventually helped me cope with daily functions.

EMDR worked so well that I would walk in my therapist's office each session with a list of 10 new issues I wanted to address. It became a joke with her because I was a typical radio reporter. We would joke that I was a "Let's get this done in 30 seconds" kind of person. She would laugh and say, "Wow, we blew through your ten items all in one session." Little did she know I had many more issues under my belt. One evening I couldn't figure out how to get out of the tub. My left leg still needed to be strengthened. My mom and I panicked, trying to figure out what to do. As I lay there, shivering in the tepid water, all I could think was, "Oh my God, the paramedics are going to see me naked!", at my next session, we had to work on bathtub anxiety. I still bring a phone in the bathroom with me for fear something unexpected may happen.

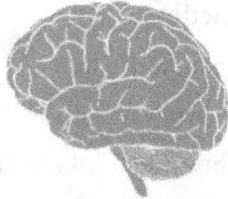

CHAPTER 26

Catherine's Gift

They say everything happens for a reason. I never had boyfriends in junior high except when I had a huge crush on Brad Jones at Hadley Junior High, but that didn't work out. Then high school was silly: my girlfriends and I would pile into "The BUE," my parents' blue Chevy. As the oldest in the group, I was always the driver, and I would choose our destination. It was always my crush's house. Around and around we would drive, giggling and singing the latest songs from the recent film *Flashdance*. I thought the words were "Take your pants off make it happen" when it was really "Take your passion and make it happen," which, incidentally, is what I am doing now. (Anyway, so what if I got the lyrics wrong? I was the driver in many ways.)

Back to boys: there were none for me. My angle changed though. Sometime during high school, I decided that I wanted to be a reporter. I liked sports and who played sports? Boys! So I went into sports reporting until some redheaded goofball, a classmate, told me I could not write for the Glen Ellyn News because I was a girl. I proclaimed to him, Guess what, I will sue the newspaper! My dad grabbed his chest and said, "You said what?!" (I thought my dad would be proud: he studied sports broadcast in college.) I told him not to worry, and I got the job anyway. But I didn't get any dates with boys.

Years later, I bought a home in Wheaton thinking a nice guy would see I was a catch and would want to date me and eventually propose. Meeting Prince Charming turned out to be not so easy. I tried lots of tricks, including online dating, praying, and changing my hair color many times. I even tried moving to Ohio for a guy, but that didn't work out either. After the aneurysm, I eventually tried dating again, but it was hard dating with a handicap placard and a cane.

Once, I convinced my physical therapist to let me go on a date without my cane. My trick was to prop myself on a chair or at a table with my legs crossed and wait for my date. That way, I didn't disclose my limp. For this date, I sat at a table during looking styling with no cane and no brace. When Larry arrived, he suggested we take a table by the door. I said Ok, hopped off my chair, and fell flat on my face. Larry turned around, picked me up and said, "Oh my God, what just happened?" We both laughed so hard. I told him the story. He said I should have told him. I told him I was embarrassed, and we laughed it off. He is still my Facebook friend. I found myself spending a lot of my life trying to hide my disability while dating. There was this goofball who asked me point blank, "What's up with the limp?" and others who were not a good fit anyway. My brain aneurysm doesn't define me; it's just something that happened to me.

After moving back to Chicago, I became fully involved in the Brain Aneurysm Foundation. On June 9, 2009, WGN TV featured me on the evening news. Just a few days later, a former Chicago paramedic asked if he could introduce me to his brother, Kevin Madden. In one of our first phone conversations, I found out that Kevin's mom, Catherine, had died on March 20, 1999 of a brain aneurysm: almost exactly five years before my rupture. He worked in the neuro intervention unit in a local hospital, and he was fascinated by my story. Our first conversation lasted 14 hours!

During our long courtship, we spent a lot of time on brain aneurysm awareness initiatives. It became our passion. During that time, for five years, Kevin and I drove to Washington, D.C. every year to lobby with the Foundation to push for federal research funding. We also worked hard on local campaigns for charity walks and cocktail parties. We helped raise $15,000 for a research chair in the BAF in honor of my Uncle Robert Sutherland who died of cancer.

Currently, both the Madden and Sutherland families support the Brain Aneurysm Foundation by volunteering at walks, lobbying, and fundraising. We believe that Catherine, in her death, brought Kevin and me together.

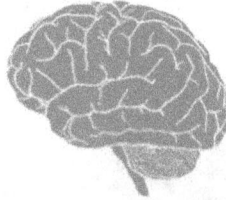

CHAPTER 27

Our Wedding

I never thought I would be marrying the man who made me so incredibly happy at 52! Geesh it took so long!! There was a funny line in the TV show *Sex and The City:* "Where is he?!" I know, right? Well, I figured, I would brand myself as a saucy blinged-up journalist but with the brain aneurysm that put a major wrench in my brand. Yeah, I have a brace, a limp, and a cane. So I had to tweak the brand. I was searching for a rare type of guy: a man who I didn't think existed. Kind, compassionate, caring, sympathetic but fun, masculine, funny, smart ass, successful, rugged, a family guy, has lots of friends, and is a little older than me. Yep, he doesn't exist, I figured. Well, when Kevin and I met at this little restaurant in the South Loop, he had white hair and smoky blue eyes. I had decided I wouldn't hide anything from him, so I showed up with my shoe cast thinking, Ok if this guy digs me, he's in. He felt bad for me. Good, there will be lots of shoe casts in the future. Buckle up, I'm a klutz! We dated for eight years. It was awesome: he was with me lobbying, at fundraisers, on fun trips, with death of our rescue dog Andrew J., family holidays. The rest is history!

My friend Katie arrived a day before the wedding to calm me down, and we drove around to find shoes to match her orange dress. So, that took a while. A couple of us ran up and down the street in Glen Ellyn and I yelled, "I am getting married, I'm an old bride!" We had a family dinner and a rehearsal dinner, after which Katie tucked me in at the hotel. The day of the wedding my friends made sure I ate because I was a nervous wreck. I got into the limo with my parents. My mom and dad's eyes got big seeing me.

We arrived at the flower-filled church and I made sure a bagpiper was playing out front for my dad, who's Scottish. We snuck into the church. All the bridesmaids were dressed in their tiffany blue dresses. My dad was nervous; he went over everything with me several times to make sure he knew what he was doing, but he was a pro! I was finally getting married, his only daughter. When we were told it was time, I started to panic. My friend who was standing nearby told me to stop and take a deep breath. I stood at the back of the church and watched my friends walk down the aisle. I was blocked from Kevin's view because I didn't want him to see me. I opted not to use my cane as I walked down the aisle with my Dad.

The church was filled with radio friends and colleagues, our families, my friends from college and our high school friends, brain aneurysm survivors, family from Ireland, my neurosurgeon, and the head of the Brain Aneurysm Foundation. It was very special to have our great friend Jan, a top radio journalist, sing at our wedding. Everyone cried as we walked down the aisle, it was such a bittersweet moment with six bridesmaids, two flower girls, and four more great nieces and nephews.

We were blessed to have Minister Arlicia Albert, herself a brain aneurysm survivor, speak at our wedding: she said, "The minute I heard Janet say, "Hey my diva girl," something inside of me stood up. Janet and I developed a strong sister bond: we have shared our secrets, our wants and desires; we have laughed together and cried together, we have shopped, we have gossiped together, we have prayed together and we have wondered what in the world has taken Kevin so long to pop the question!"

Guests were greeted at the reception with the bagpiper, and an Irish band played all night long. My brother Mark welcomed Kevin into the family with a toast: "Thank you for making Janet so happy. We know you are taking great care of her and that's a really big deal." My maid of honor, Becky, in her toast, said, "Janet is like Swarovski crystal and Kevin is the one that keeps her polished and shining."

Life is beautiful. June 17, 2017

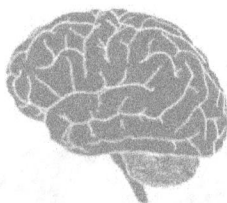

CHAPTER 28

Things I Have Learned

I may seem 100 percent now but I am not.

The up side is, I have learned so much about my body. It has completely changed and reacts to things differently than it did before the rupture. Once you have a craniotomy, there is a one in five chance that you will have a seizure. The seizures are caused by scar tissues in the brain. Often they are brought on by stress or dehydration. I have been having seizures since the time I met my husband Kevin. I've passed out in the heat due to lack of water. I have panic attacks in airplanes and on heights, which cause me to turn white and nearly pass out. I am constantly aware of my limp and always try, unsuccessfully, to hide it from people. When I walk, people stare at my leg rather than looking at my face first. I use a handicap placard in my car, and although it gets me a great parking space at the mall, other shoppers can be cruel. Some have commented to me, "You don't look handicapped," so be prepared for that. I know when it's going to snow or rain because my head hurts. I fall a lot due to my weak leg and have ended up in the ER many times. My poor balance inhibits many activities.

Unfortunately, my weak left side and "suck it up" attitude have caused me to take unnecessary risks. In 2016, my job in marketing demanded that I lift heavy boxes, walk up and down stairs, and stand a lot on the job. Not being able to feel my left foot, I was unaware when I developed a stress fracture in that foot. It was the swelling that alerted me. As recently as one year ago, I got angry because I was told I could not ride a bike. No one told me why so I got on the bike and rode with one foot. I fell off the bike backwards. I fell directly on my head, suffered a concussion and suffered some minor deficits.

Many brain aneurysm survivors refuse to take antidepressants but others of us have found them very helpful. I finally started taking antidepressants 12 years after my aneurysm. I wish I had taken them when my doctor prescribed them; it would have saved me much hysteria. I feel like I am still recovering from my brain aneurysm.

According to Deidre A. Buckley, nurse practitioner and past president of the Brain Aneurysm Foundation Board of

Directors, recover y from a burst brain aneurysm depends on several things: its location in the brain, its size and the type of rupture. The blood that spills erases patterns in the brain. That's why I needed to relearn how to walk. How long might it take someone else to transition from a wheelchair to a walker to a cane and then to walking without any help? It depends on the individual. There may be numerous challenges as you heal. For me, there was the lack of vision. Once I had the surgery to restore some vision, I was able to work on strengthening my stomach and back muscles to use a walker. Many other muscles were weakened, and I had no idea how much I depended on them: hip, bladder, vaginal, thigh, and the list goes on.

Once I was able to get my lower half semi-strong enough to use a walker, I learned how to transition from a sitting position to standing at the walker. I leaned forward and then put my nose over toes, pushing off over my knees and using the walker slowly. Heel to the toe, heel to the toe. I was laying the brain patterns back down again, retraining my brain how to walk again, how to sit, how to do everything. So, especially at first, each day was exhausting because my brain was busy learning every day. Because I could not and still cannot feel my left foot, I have learned to be careful to watch it. Not a day goes by that I am not glancing down, making sure my foot is straight and not sticking out to the side. Every day is a challenge and I never stop thinking when I walk or sit or step over a curb.

Therefore, because everyone is different, there is no formula for how long recovery takes. Don't let your doctor tell you two months; you will watch the calendar and wait for two months and you may feel the same. I did that and was disappointed. It may be six months or two weeks, who knows?! You may have a trachea hole in your throat or a dent in your head; you may have neither of those things. I have both. You may not be able to speak or your speaking may be fine. Your aneurysm may have been coiled and there may not have been any craniotomy and you went home in a week. I was in the hospital for four months, blind for seven months, paralyzed on my left side for four months, and I still go to physical therapy. We survivors must simply give it time: work hard at therapy, be patient, pray, hope for the best, and prepare for the worst. I was given a three percent chance to live and could have been in a vegetative state. I have a friend who survived a brain aneurysm but died of a stroke years later. The best course is to embrace life and fight for others.

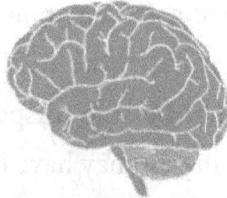

CHAPTER 29

Lobbying For Awareness

Education to first responders can save lives. On March 22, 2004 Norwich Township Fire Department paramedics responded to my apartment after hearing the dispatcher say that I had the "worst head-ache ever." According to firefighter Jason Fisher, "That was a big red flag that we need to get moving." He knew that I was in pretty bad shape, and the fact that I was having seizures and vomiting meant "we needed to get you into the truck to go to the hospital to get a CT scan." The ambulance ran full lights and sirens and the paramedics worked to stabilize me, to get me breathing and relaxed to Doctors West Hospital.

When I decided that I wanted to increase awareness across the country, I realized that it was a daunting task. I have been hesitant to step into the spotlight about my brain aneurysm, not knowing if people will look at me differently, and they have. However, I am compelled to use my past illness to encourage survivors and caregivers to never give up and to support the Brain Aneurysm Foundation. There are laws that can protect you; I am alive and grateful to tell you about my journey.

For the last six years, the Brain Aneurysm Foundation has traveled to the Capitol seeking research funding and awareness for brain aneurysms. My husband and I have joined them each spring. Every year, we meet hundreds of survivors, many of whom bring their family members. In sharing our stories, it is interesting to learn that many of us were professional women, driven and focused on our careers. We should have been alarmed by the intensity of the headaches we all experienced rather than considering them just a nuisance. It was an annoyance to stop work and get checked for what we thought was simply a bad headache.

Although our situations are all different, we share common denominators: the fear that we had almost died, the nagging question of if it could happen again, memory issues, and an observation of the lack of public awareness. Those are the reasons why we are all in Washington D.C, even though the journey and effort were quite fatiguing. The first year, I was one of the few using a cane; most others were in wheelchairs.

Other people lobby because they have lost children or other family members to brain aneurysms They are fueled by grief, and it is our honor to work side by side with them. When we lobby, Kevin and I are doing it for survivors in Illinois, and we are remembering those who are like his parents.

At the start of lobby day, we meet in the morning with the legal firm who oversees the lobbying initiative. We are typically scheduled for eleven meetings. Our packets are full of information about brain aneurysms and statistics as to how much research funding we want. If we cannot meet directly with the senators and congressmen, we leave these packets with their aides. We are determined to walk in the heavy, sweltering, soaking heat through the halls of Congress, to keep our appointments and make our pitches. I turn on my brace that has an electric stimulation (so I am shocking myself) in order to demonstrate the need for research and to push for more funding and awareness. I hobble up and down the hallways with blisters on my feet, sometimes meeting with an aide in the hallway; we do what we must, so long as we got our message out. The 10 years I have in sales have served me well: I am used to knocking on doors. Sometimes we race across streets from our cabs in order to make our appointments. The DC cops would yell at me, but I yelled back! This is literally a life and death mission we are on. My husband Kevin continues to support me in this mission, as have many life-long friends: my junior high friend Barry Holmes traveled from Kansas to support me in DC.

I am reminded of what former Ohio State University Football Coach Woody Hayes said: "You can never really pay back. You can only pay forward." Since moving back to Chicago, I have begun to "pay forward" in Illinois. In April 2007, the Illinois House passed a bill making September Brain Aneurysm Awareness Month. The bill was sponsored by former State Representative Sandra Pihos. At least half a dozen states are currently working on awareness legislation.

"Let us not look back in anger, nor forward in fear, but around us in awareness." James Thurber

EPILOGUE

A Tribute to a Man's Man

The little guy, just a wide-eyed tot, was perhaps four or five years old the first time he saw a baseball game at sleepy old Griffith Stadium in Washington D.C. He was in awe, enthralled and boyishly energized by what took place on the diamond with his beloved Washington Senators and the indomitable Walter "Big Train" Johnson. The "Train" was beyond one-of-a-kind: he was simply the greatest right-handed pitcher in major league baseball history. While winning 417 games, he also racked up 110 career shutouts and established several records that have lasted since Al Capone was the unofficial mayor of Chicago.

Our little guy eventually gravitated up the coast to Millburn, New Jersey where his heart-rooting interest would switch to the colorful Brooklyn Dodgers. He was a book of knowledge on the historic "Boys of Summer": Jackie, Duke, Carl Furillo, Newk, Campy and the other tough guys from Flatbush.

However, his heart would finds its rightful spot in 1974 when he moved his family to Chicago and established a non-stop love affair with the Cubs. My God, he endured highs and lows with the "Loveable Losers," but his loyalty, much like his devotion to his family and all things he believed to be honorable, would never waver. Our guy lived and died with the Cubbies. He held on to every word from Hall of Fame broadcasters Jack Brickhouse and Harry Caray.

This man, who packed a 212-degree wallop of friendship, was nothing if not genuine.

You see, Donald Ripley "Don" Sutherland was worthy of being described as a man's man. His was the hand that would help, the heart that would comfort, the soothing words that would bring joy out of sadness.

Don has left us. I would like to think he's sipping a cold beer while talking baseball with long gone Cubs like Hack Wilson and "Three Finger" Brown. Whatever the case may be: Don, you were the life of a wonderful party. You will never be forgotten by those who were blessed to know you.

I don't say that casually or to be proper. I'm simply speaking the truth. Don, find the "Big Train." Engage him in hot stove baseball gossip. I know Mr. Johnson will appreciate your Knowledge, and of far greater importance - your class.

Chet Coppock

7/11/18

Chet Coppock and Don Sutherland both shared a passion for baseball and worked together on a fundraiser for the Brain Aneurysm Foundation at a minor league baseball game at the Gary Railcats.

Chet Coppock has done national TV commercials for Wheaties with the late Walter Payton. For ten years, he teamed up with Michael Jordan as the Voice of Chicagoland and Northwest Indiana Chevrolet. For nine years, Coppock served as a sportscaster on WISH TV (CBS) in Indianapolis and WMAQ TV (NBC) in Chicago. And for three years, he hosted *NewSport Talk*, a New York-based live TV interview and call-in show carried by Cablevision.

APPENDIX A

Janet's Advice

According to Dr. Sepideh Amin-Hanjani, MD, FAANS, FACS, FAHA, Brain Aneurysm Foundation medical advisor board member, Professor, Residency Program Director, Co-Director of Neurovascular Surgery, University of Illinois at Chicago, "between 20-30% of people with ruptured aneurysms have multiple aneurysms at the time of presentation." Little was known about brain aneurysms when I was being treated. According to Hanjani, "New aneurysms can develop even after existing aneurysms (are) treated."

Here's what I advise:

- Make sure you understand the ADA & HIPPA law.
- Try not to share too many of the details of your brain aneurysm with your employer; discrimination may occur, no matter who they are, even if your employer seems to be supportive. #MeToo
- Don't go back to work too soon, you will be tired and confused and the office lights may bother you and if you make a mistake you may lose your confidence.

- You will have headaches when it rains or snows. Talk to your neurologist when this happens.
- You will blame every mistake on your brain aneurysm. Remember, you are human.
- It's okay to be mad at God; seek pastoral counseling.
- Take advantage of social security disability, there's no shame on going on disability; get a lawyer if you need to.
- If you have short or long-term disability insurance with your employer, use it.
- Make sure you have all legal documents ready like power of attorney etc.
- Expect some of your relationships to change; it's not you, it's them.
- Find out if there is a history of brain aneurysms in your family; if so talk to your doctor.
- Look for a local brain aneurysm support group and attend it if you can; it will be very helpful.
- Lean on the Brain Aneurysm Foundation as a resource- www.bafound.org

After spending four months in a rehabilitation hospital to transition from a wheelchair to a walker, I was discharged home and then went to outpatient rehabilitation. It took months and months until I was able to use a cane. Everyone is different. The Brain Aneurysm Foundation helped me transition home and back into my new life. The Foundation created brochures focusing on the various topics most survivors one will face. I faced all of them.

I can't begin to stress how important it is to discharge brain aneurysm patients with information about their condition. Their families need this information as well. I have worked with the Brain Aneurysm Foundation and area hospitals to create discharge packets. Much of the following information is in those packets.

APPENDIX B

The Brain Aneurysm Foundation

Founded in Boston and now based in Hanover, Massachusetts, the Brain Aneurysm Foundation is the globally recognized leader in brain aneurysm awareness, education, support, advocacy and research funding. To date the foundation is the largest private funder of brain aneurysm research.

The foundation's mission is to provide information about and raise awareness of the symptoms and risk factors of brain aneurysms to prevent ruptures and subsequent death and disability; work with medical communities to provide support networks for patients and families; and advance research to improve patients' outcomes and save lives.

Established in 1994, the foundation has a Medical Advisory Board that comprises more than 30 of the nation's foremost aneurysm experts — neurologists, neurosurgeons, interventional neuroradiologists and other brain aneurysm specialists — from the country's leading hospitals and universities.

With 1 in 50 people walking around with a brain aneurysm, 30,000 people a year rupturing and half of these people dying, there is still much to be done for awareness and education. www.bafound.org

APPENDIX C

For Survivors

The Brain Aneurysm Foundation has some helpful advice for survivors. Nurse Practitioner Deidra Buckley encourages caregivers and survivors to utilize **the following information that is also available on the foundation's website** to help in the recovery process.

After Your Treatment

You can expect some changes in the first few days and weeks following your treatment. Which of these you experience and how long they last depends on a number of factors, including whether your aneurysm had ruptured prior to treatment and the type of treatment (open or endovascular) you had.

Open Surgery
Issues after open surgery (clipping) may include:

- **Incision Pain/Numbness** The pain usually occurs at the incision site. It may take several weeks for the incision to heal. After this time, you may experience brief episodes of sharp pain in the incision area as the nerves grow back.

This is not cause for concern. The pain will go away with time. The incision area can also feel numb; this may or may not get better with time. It may be uncomfortable to sleep on the side with the incision, but it is safe to do so.

- **Hearing Loss** You may notice muffled hearing in the ear on the same side as the incision. This is due to fluid accumulation and will get better with time. However, it may take several weeks to notice improvement.

- **Jaw Pain** may occur when you open your mouth to eat or brush your teeth. This is due to manipulation of the muscles during surgery. The pain will improve over time. You may be able to speed up your recovery by opening and closing your mouth (about 10 times) at least four to five times a day, gradually increasing how wide you open it. Let your surgeon know if the pain persists after six weeks; in this case, physical therapy may be advised.

- **Clicking Noise in Head** commonly occurs when you position your head in different ways. While alarming, there is no need to be concerned. This is the bone healing and a normal part of the recovery process. The clicking goes away after several weeks.

- **Seizures** may occur at the time of aneurysm rupture or sometimes as a result of surgery on certain parts of the brain. Your neurosurgeon may put you on an anti-seizure medication in the hospital. In certain cases your doctor will have you continue this medicine after you go home. If there are no further seizures, the medicine is usually continued for only a short time. If you are on anti-seizure medicine, it is important that you take the medicine as prescribed.

- Endovascular Treatment Issues

After endovascular treatment (also called embolization), symptoms may include groin pain: there may be bruising and discomfort where the catheter was inserted in the groin. You should avoid strenuous activity and hot baths for one week after treatment. A hematoma (hard large blood clot) can develop at the site. Should this happen, or if there is increased pain or swelling in the area, contact the doctor who performed the procedure. Another symptom might be hair loss due to radiation or the contrast dye used during the procedure. This usually only affects a small area and is temporary — the hair will grow back. Keep in mind that stress and medicines can also cause temporary hair loss.

- Attention and Executive Function

Most survivors have problems focusing. Their attention span is short. They start something but do not finish it and find their attention drifting from one thing to another. They get easily flustered when they try to shop, for example. Some of this may be due to fatigue and is another reason why rest is so important. However, the main reason is that the brain is still trying to heal itself and is not yet functioning normally. In this situation, the brain cannot do too much at one time.

Executive Function: Living the most fulfilling life possible requires juggling multiple goals, making complex decisions, and solving problems that life invariably creates. Most survivors find it challenging to return to optimal functioning, which requires carrying out this juggling act flawlessly while achieving goals and removing obstacles. Many find themselves struggling to know what to do first, how to organize their day or goals, or find ways to get themselves unstuck. Some experience a sense of being overwhelmed, in addition to poor motivation and general lethargy, making it difficult to get through the day. Finally, some may notice a general impulsivity when doing work that requires careful evaluation and comparison of options. Here are some tips to help you focus and improve your executive function:

- Break up projects into short mini-projects.
- Make a daily schedule of activities and stick to it as much as possible.
- Have a family member assist with projects and help you remember to focus.
- Seek out a quiet room if necessary.
- Avoid noise and lots of people, as this can be overwhelming. Instead, participate in quiet, enjoyable, one-on-one activities such as going for a walk with a

friend or out to dinner at a quiet restaurant with a family member. Avoid busy places like malls.

- Do not try to do too much at one time. For instance, do not try to simultaneously watch TV, do a crossword puzzle, and talk on the phone.

Memory

Memory involves many parts of the brain, and if a brain aneurysm rupture or treatment damages any of those areas, your memory will be affected. Survivors of ruptured aneurysms usually do not remember the event or much of what happened in the hospital, and never will. This can be disconcerting but is normal. Many survivors regain their ability to remember as they continue to heal, while some continue to have difficulty with short-term or working memory for years. Survivors might remember events from ten years ago but cannot seem to remember who called yesterday or where they put their keys. Absorbing, storing, and recalling information are some of the challenges survivors face after a rupture or treatment of a brain aneurysm. Learning new material in general may be difficult. Some have difficulty with something called prospective memory, which is the ability to remember future events. Here are several strategies for coping with these issues.

To help absorb information:

- Link — associate new information with old information.
- Simplify — avoid sensory and language overload. Shorten sentences for easier understanding; break up large pieces of information in order to focus better.
- Use apps that help with memory or record new information on your smartphone. Write down notes or memos to help jog your memory.

To help store information:

- Repeat and rehearse — immediately after someone says something or you learn something new, repeat it to yourself. Then wait a few minutes, and repeat it again to see if you remember.

Support Groups

Being diagnosed with or treated for a brain aneurysm is a life-changing experience. Many survivors and their loved ones benefit from ongoing support through attendance at monthly support groups. The Brain Aneurysm Foundation started the first support group in Boston in 1992. Since then, the foundation has worked with healthcare providers across the United States and Canada to establish more than 60 support groups. Support groups, which are typically held monthly and led by healthcare professionals, help by:

- Letting survivors and loved ones know they are not alone and that others understand what they are going through.
- Providing a confidential setting where members can share emotions, experiences, and challenges with others in similar circumstances.
- Providing a forum for solving problems and sharing ideas.
- Providing reliable health information, reasonable expectations for recovery, and resources.
- Enabling healthcare professionals to educate patients — and for patients to educate healthcare professionals about their experiences.
- Helping patients find appropriate resources. A list of Brain Aneurysm Foundation-approved support groups is on our website (bafound.org). If you are a healthcare professional interested in organizing a support group in your area, contact the Brain Aneurysm Foundation, which will assist you.

Individual Psychotherapy

Brain aneurysm survivors can face a number of challenges: as mentioned previously, difficulties with anxiety, depression, and lack of confidence and self-esteem are not uncommon. While some survivors return to their previous level of functioning, others may be adapting to the "new normal" in their lives. In this situation, individual psychotherapy can be a valuable component of your return to good health. In many states in the United States, mental health services are covered by medical insurance. Your primary care doctor and/or your neurosurgeon can provide a referral. Insurance companies maintain an online list of mental health providers in your area.

APPENDIX D

Physical Challenges

Recovery for patients who receive treatment for an unruptured aneurysm generally requires less rehabilitative therapy and those patients recover more quickly than patients whose aneurysm has ruptured. Recovery from treatment or rupture may take weeks to months.

During the recovery process, whether at the beginning or two years from your last surgery, you might experience some unusual physical challenges. It is comforting to know that you are not alone and that many brain aneurysm survivors are facing similar experiences. Most of these challenges will fade into the background as time goes by, while others will remain constant for many years, depending on your particular situation. Patience and time are your two best allies to the success of your recovery.

Recovery from a ruptured brain aneurysm is influenced by many factors. The most important factor is the patient's clinical condition on admission based on the extent of the initial hemorrhage. Some patients are devastated neurologically from the time of rupture. Others do surprisingly well.

Headaches

Most patients experience different levels of headaches depending on the severity of the aneurysm, whether it ruptured, as well as the type of treatment. Many times, patients who have a hemorrhage will develop a secondary migraine condition as a result of the injury. Headaches can last for two weeks or two years, depending on these variables, as well as change of seasons, health, and stress. Headaches can bring about fear and concern. You might worry that you have another aneurysm or wonder if you could have another hemorrhage. Your chances of re-rupture are low, almost zero. However, there are rare instances when new aneurysms may grow or rupture. If you have the second "worst headache of your life," seek medical attention.

Drowsiness and Fatigue

Exhaustion is a very common complaint from brain aneurysm survivors. This can last for months, even years. The brain takes a very long time to heal, and the energy required for the healing process to take place is great. Also, some of the medications you might be taking could be causing you to feel sluggish and require frequent napping. Napping is good and is helping your body heal. Listen to your body, and rest as needed.

Incision Pain

This pain is usually localized to the surgical site. It may take several weeks to heal, and in some cases, absence of touch sensation may not fully return. It may be uncomfortable to sleep on the side that has the incision. However, it is okay to do this without doing any damage.

Balance and Coordination

After SAH there may be problems with balance and coordination.

Jaw Pain and Speech Impairment

Most common on the operative side of the face, and occurs when you try to open your mouth to eat or brush your teeth. To speed up the healing process, exercise your jaw by opening and closing your mouth (about ten times) as wide as you can at least four to five times per day. Notify your doctor, if the jaw pain persists for more than six weeks. After rupture, and depending on location of SAH, a patient may experience difficulty with speech and swallowing.

Clicking Noise (Head)

You might hear a clicking noise, almost sounding like metal rubbing together. This is common when you position your head in different ways and can be alarming. There is no need to panic. It is actually the bone healing and will take a long time to stop.

Back Pain

Because you may have been confined to bed for a long period of time, you may have lost muscle mass, coordination, and balance. Some patients experience sciatica, a shooting pain down the back of your leg, as a result of this lack of activity, and will require physical therapy. Stretching exercises or a heating pad will help alleviate this pain.

Hair Loss

Some medications, the dye from the angiogram, as well as stress, may cause initial hair loss. Do not be alarmed, it will grow back.

Constipation

This may be an issue due to lack of mobility and addition of pain medication. You may need to take a soft laxative, such as Metamucil, or a stool softener, like Colace. Do not strain or push too hard!

Hearing Loss

Fluid might have accumulated in your ears and takes several weeks to disappear, making hearing on the side of the surgery diminished. This will improve in time, generally over a period of weeks.

Vision Problems

Depending on aneurysm location, you may experience blurred, double, or peripheral vision problems. Consult with your physician.

Decreased Fine Motor Control

Will return in most cases.

Delayed Menstruation

Is common. Talk to your gynecologist.

Weight Gain or Weight Loss

May be medication-related or due to lack of activity

Seizures

A seizure is caused by abnormal electrical activity in the brain. Seizures may consist of strange sensations, blackouts, jerking in the arms and legs, lapses of consciousness, or a combination of these symptoms.

If you had a hemorrhage from your aneurysm, you will most likely be on seizure medication for a short time. It is important for you to monitor yourself for seizure activity, although your chances of having one are minimal, due to taking an anticonvulsant. Most unruptured aneurysm patients do not take seizure medication unless specified by their neurosurgeon.

After treatment, most patients will spend a couple days in the Intensive Care Unit. He/she will be closely monitored for pressure on the brain, any new bleeding, threat of vasospasm, as well as making sure all other body functions are working properly.

If you are on an anticonvulsant, you will probably remain on this medication for several weeks to months, or until the risk of further seizures is gone. You or a family member should make sure you take the medication on a regular basis. Depending on the medication, your doctor will draw blood frequently to determine appropriate drug levels for this medication.

If you are experiencing postoperative seizures, you must surrender your driver's license to the Registry (Department) of Motor Vehicles. You or your doctor will contact the RMV/DMV after the seizures are gone.

Do not drink alcohol while taking this medication. Alcohol lowers your threshold for seizure activity, and may cause further complications.

APPENDIX E

Emotional Challenges

No one can truly know what you are feeling or what you have gone through, because each experience is unique. However, other survivors have had some or all of the following emotional experiences, during their recovery. Brain aneurysms, hemorrhage, and brain surgery are traumatic occurrences. Whether it is the lack of memory of the incident that is scaring you, or concerns for your future capabilities, you have been through a life-altering experience. It is okay to be frightened, but know, that you are not alone. There are people who want to help you, support you, and listen.

An important part of the recovery process and healing is maintaining a positive mindset. The patient needs to stay focused on healing, being positive, maintaining a healthy diet, getting back to exercise as allowed by the physician, and being with friends and family.

Depression

This is very common to all survivors, whether you suffered a ruptured aneurysm or were treated for an unruptured aneurysm. Some of it may be chemical, while another part may be physical. Going through this type of illness can be a traumatic and life-changing event for many people. It can bring about positive and negative changes in people, and many times depression results from this. There is no need to suffer in silence.

Depression is an illness that involves the body, mood, and thoughts. It affects the way a person eats and sleeps, the way one feels about oneself, and the way one thinks about life. It is not simply a passing blue mood or a sudden feeling of sadness that goes away as quickly as it came.

Many brain aneurysm survivors suffer from depression as a result of this traumatic event. Because one's lifestyle has been changed, and the ability to do things they used to be able to do has changed, feelings of helplessness and hopelessness can occur. Treatment, a combination of medication and therapy, can help survivors deal with depression and feel better.

You and your family should advocate for neurological testing by a neuropsychiatrist. If not that, you should make every effort to see a neuropsychologist who can help you deal with the depression. They can determine what the best course of treatment is, recommend therapists, and help you conquer this sadness.

Survivors who exhibit some or all of these symptoms should seek help:

- Mood swings

- Constant feelings of sadness, anxiousness, or emptiness
- Pessimistic outlook on life
- Feelings of hopelessness
- Decreased energy and fatigue
- Difficulty concentrating
- Unable to make decisions
- Forgetfulness
- Insomnia or sleeping too much
- Appetite and weight changes
- Loss of interest or pleasure in activities, including sex
- Physical ailments, like headaches and digestive problems
- Suicidal thoughts

You need to openly share your concerns and your feelings with someone close to you as well as with a medical professional that understands your condition. Having to depend on others during your recovery and losing a sense of independence can interfere with your confidence, but know that it does get better over time.

Your daily life may be affected by mental and physical fatigability. Intolerance to being rushed, to groups of people, to small children, to lack of order or routine, and to normal sound levels are common complaints. It is difficult to measure these problems objectively, and they can compromise personal relationships and employment. Family relationships may suffer, and intimate relationships may be affected by lack of libido. Patience and time are your two best allies to the success of your recovery. No one should suffer alone, so seek help.

Loss of Emotional Control

Most survivors experience temporary loss of control over emotions. In some cases, the brain has been injured, and this can cause some changes to a person's emotional state. This can manifest itself in anger, frustration, and lashing out at oneself and others. Confusion about the trauma is common, so talk about it to your family and friends. If it becomes too difficult to deal with it alone, seek counseling.

Lowered Self-Esteem

Changes in your self-image and self-confidence as a result of new physical and mental limitations may occur. You need to talk to your family, doctor, and therapist about how you feel and how to deal with the "new" you. You are not any less capable of leading a normal life. It is just going to take adjusting to your surroundings and time to heal.

Insomnia or Difficulty Sleeping

Many survivors voice concerns about changes in their sleeping patterns. Some people sleep all day, while others do not sleep at all. There could be many reasons why sleep has been affected, both emotional and physical reasons. You should talk to your doctor if you are having trouble sleeping, especially if it becomes a real problem.

Relationship Issues — for you, your family, and your friends.

Loneliness — feeling different, being isolated for long periods of time.

APPENDIX F

Potential Deficits

Survivors of brain aneurysms might suffer short-term and/or long-term deficits as a result of a rupture or treatment. In thirty percent of the cases, these deficits disappear over time.

The recovery process is long and it takes weeks, months, and maybe years to understand the level of deficits you incurred as a result of this trauma.

Survivors should seek neurological assessment from a neuropsychiatrist or neuropsychologist to determine the level of cognitive functioning and associated problems. In many cases, patients enlist speech, physical, and occupational therapists to help them regain normal functions.

For subarachnoid hemorrhage (SAH) survivors, the deficits are often greater, more noticeable, and require a longer recovery period. Some, not all, SAH and unruptured aneurysm survivors suffer from the following:

- Stroke (mainly SAH)
- Partial or complete blindness (mainly SAH)
- Peripheral vision deficits (both)
- Cognitive processing problems (both)

- Speech complications (both)
- Perceptual problems (both)
- Behavioral inconsistencies (both)
- Loss of balance and coordination (Posterior circulation aneurysms)
- Decreased concentration (both)
- Short-term memory difficulties (both)
- Fatigue (both)

Most of these deficits decrease over time with healing and therapy. Many stroke victims recover with increased therapy and regain most of their functions. More severe hemorrhagic patients might suffer more serious and longer effects. Each patient has a unique set of difficulties.

Work with family members to help you notice your strengths and weaknesses. Sometimes, they are the best ones to notice what slight deficits you might have. They can help be your eyes and ears, as well as help you gain a better understanding of how to deal with these subtle differences. Many of the "background" deficits that are subtler tend to last longer, making it difficult for survivors. Be patient with yourself, and talk to your therapist or doctor about how to deal with these subtle difficulties.

APPENDIX G

What To Expect

Rehabilitation and Recovery

The families of brain aneurysm survivors may need to make difficult decisions and deal with extremely challenging circumstances. Changes in behavior, mood and emotions are common after surgery. Some patients also may experience deficits in cognitive, or thinking, abilities. Such changes present challenges for caregivers trying to help the patient recover. The caregiver is crucial to successful rehabilitation, so learning everything about the aneurysm and its effects on behavior as well as physical function will help you respond effectively. It is important to remember that these changes are caused by the aneurysm itself, and not the patient. The rehabilitation of the ruptured aneurysm patient requires strong and loving support from the family, as well as a quality rehabilitation team of doctors and therapists to optimize the patient's recovery from the devastation caused by a brain aneurysm.

Information sources

Your doctor, nurse practitioner, or case manager are all excellent sources to help you explore various rehabilitation options. Websites and support groups dedicated to brain aneurysms also are useful. Perhaps the best sources are patients who have successfully undergone surgery and caregivers who have helped them resume their daily lives.

Paths to recovery

In the best-case scenario, patient and caregiver know about the aneurysm in advance and make decisions about rehabilitation before surgery. A planned surgery typically creates mild-to-moderate cognitive and physical issues. The recovery period for elective treatment in patients with an unruptured aneurysm is usually shorter and less complex than for an emergency treatment in patients with a ruptured aneurysm.

A more serious situation occurs when an aneurysm unexpectedly ruptures and leads to emergency surgery. The physical and psychological effects from unplanned emergency surgery can be more serious because the aneurysm has already ruptured and caused damage to brain tissue. Moderate-to-severe cognitive and physical limitations may result. Fatigue and weakness can persist for a few months after hospitalization. New physical impairments after **subarachnoid hemorrhage (SAH)** include wound related discomfort, problems with balance and coordination, weakness in one or more limbs, difficulty with speech and swallowing and problems with vision. Over time these deficits may improve partially or entirely. Physically, healing may take months to a few years.

APPENDIX H

For Caregivers: Dealing With Emotional Distress

It is not unusual for a family member to experience emotional distress at any phase of the rehabilitation process. Often, the family member is unaware of the distress because the primary focus is always on the survivor's needs. You, the caregiver, are also in need of professional help during this family crisis.

During and immediately after the aneurysm, the family of the survivor experiences a broad range of intense emotions, such as shock, fear, worry, anger, frustration, and hopelessness. As the rehabilitation process unfolds, these emotions may continue to prey on you and further add to your already suffering. Depression, worry, anger, and grief may pile on top of your own fragile emotions. You might feel guilty and brush this feeling aside because you are so anxious to take proper care of your loved one. You may find it difficult to fully express and explore your feelings if the survivor is present.

Others in your situation probably undergo the same feelings and you are not alone. The emotional distress that you may experience is a natural part of the rehabilitation process and you must realize that self-care is just as important as survivor care. Your emotional wellbeing is necessary for a positive outcome for both you and the brain aneurysm survivor.

There are many forms of emotional distress. You, the caregiver, should not view these depressed, anxious or hopeless moods as a sign of weakness. When you realize the gamut of emotions that you have experienced from the beginning of the aneurysm episode until the present, you will begin to appreciate how stressful life has been for you as well as for your loved one. It is important to release your emotions and understand the commonality of your feelings amongst caregivers.

It will be important for you to maintain a positive outlook throughout your care giving, which will help you develop patience with the survivor and the process. You will learn that personality and behavior changes after an aneurysm are generally not intentional, but reflect changes in brain function.

The way any family member interprets the survivor's behavior and progress plays a major role in his/her emotional condition. Consider the family of a survivor who has an aneurysm that affected the function of her frontal lobes. The frontal lobe has a great deal to do with initiation and motivation, and survivors with damage to this area may not take obvious steps toward recovery, and seem "lazy" or uncaring. The family of a survivor with poor motivation may become upset if they believe that the survivor has lost interest and given up. If you, as the caregiver, think that the patient is deliberately avoiding recovery work, you may become quite frustrated or angry with that survivor. If, on the other hand, you understand the neurological basis for the survivor's poor motivation, you will deal much more effectively with the problem. You will have the patience to structure the survivor's activities, and actively encourage him/her to work toward rehabilitation goals.

As the caregiver, you must remember that your emotional wellbeing is crucial to the progress of your survivor's health. You must recognize and tend to your own emotional struggles in order to be successful. If you are the primary caregiver, consider the benefits of an aneurysm support group or a caregiver support group or private therapy. It will be a safe harbor to moor your emotions during this turbulent time.

10 Tips for Caregivers

- Caregiving is a job, and respite is your earned right. **Reward yourself** with respite breaks often.
- **Watch out** for signs of depression, and don't delay in getting professional help when you need it.
- When people offer to help, **accept the offer** and suggest specific things that they can do.
- **Educate yourself** about your loved one's condition and how to communicate effectively with doctors.

- There's a difference between caring and doing. **Be open** to technologies and ideas that promote your loved one's independence.
- **Trust your instincts.** Most of the time, they'll lead you in the right direction.
- Caregivers often do the lifting, pushing, and pulling. **Be good to your back.**
- Grieve for your losses and then allow yourself to **dream new dreams.**
- **Seek support** from other caregivers. There is great strength in knowing you are not alone.
- Stand up for your rights as a caregiver and a citizen.

APPENDIX I

How Can I Help

As the caregiver, you will require many tools to assist your loved one to recover. Your education in this process is essential for your own welfare in addition to the survivor's wellbeing.

You will need to set up and execute a rehabilitation treatment plan with direction from a neuropsychologist or other trained rehabilitation professional. This information will be invaluable once the aneurysm survivor has returned home. You should be educated about how to create an ideal environment for rehabilitation progress.

You and your survivor will benefit from working systematically toward planned goals. Those who have no plan sense their lack of direction and become easily discouraged. There are a few important learning principles that you, as the caregiver, should understand:

Treatment Plan. A good treatment plan identifies problem areas and breaks these issues into manageable steps. For example, a survivor who has problems getting dressed in the morning (due to problems with decision-making, organization, and speed) can learn to select clothing and organize the process by addressing each part of the problem at a time. The most effective treatment plan involves active participation by you during the initial phases of new learning, with gradual withdrawal of support as the survivor learns new habits.

Survivor Goals. It is important for you to determine the survivor's goals from a short – term perspective, one behavior at a time. Large paces make it impossible to work on small steps. Patience is a necessary part of the process, as many failures have to be endured to achieve mastery of any skill. Remind to teach your survivor that failures are a necessary part of improvement, rather than something to be ashamed of or embarrassed about.

Positive Feedback. Progress is generally made when the survivor feels good about accomplishments. Remember to use reinforcements and rewards, to encourage step-by-step progress. Almost everyone responds well to encouragement and approval. We all shrink from angry words and harsh criticism. Punishment, sharp words, criticism, and disapproval are never effective and will only yield side effects such as anger, avoidance, and aggression. A rewarding atmosphere leads to high levels of hope and increased levels of effort.

As the caregiver, you want to see your loved one function independently and successfully. You will need to take advantage of all the support that is available to help you to reach that goal. It will take patience, kindness and persistence for you and your survivor to achieve results and you must remember that it is possible to see your loved one make great progress in their recovery.

APPENDIX J

Aids to Recovery

You will have good days and bad days, negative thoughts and positive thoughts, moments of peace and moments of turmoil. Celebrate the good days, enjoy the peaceful moments of solitude and reflection, and write down positive thoughts so you can remember them. Keep in mind that healing and recovery is a marathon, not a sprint. One key to a positive recovery is to resume your responsibilities and activities gradually, and with confidence. Although these responsibilities and activities might be different than in the past and take on a whole new meaning, they allow you to make progress and contribute to the success of your recovery. So ask yourself, "What have I always wanted to do with my time? Are there interests I want to pursue? How can I turn this situation into a positive one that makes me feel good about myself?" Keeping a journal allows you to express your feelings and develop an inner peace about your condition. Journaling is also a good way to monitor progress of certain cognitive functions, like handwriting, language, and storytelling. If you are unable to write, use a recorder or ask a friend or family member to be your "scribe." This will be therapeutic for both of you. Other ways to express your feelings are through poetry, song, painting, and meditation.

APPENDIX K

Returning to Work/School

For many people, work is an important part of their identity. In many cases, returning to work or school is an achievable goal. But how you defined work before your treatment may be different from how you define it now. Perhaps you will decide to work or return to school part time instead of full-time, for example. If you are considering returning to work or school, you will certainly have many questions. When can I return? What types of work can I do? What if I go back to work and realize I am not able to perform the same functions I once could? If I am receiving Social Security Disability Insurance, how will returning to work affect this? Are there services to help me ease into returning to work? If you decide to return to work or school and your doctor says it is okay to do so, you might face some challenges. Many people are not aware of the "background" deficits associated with brain trauma, so your employer may not understand that expecting you to perform at your previous capacity might be unrealistic. Before returning to work or school, it is important for you to be assessed by a neuropsychiatrist, neuropsychologist, or other rehabilitation professional to determine what cognitive deficits you may have, as they will impact how you function in the workplace/classroom. These deficits might include memory, organizational skills, language processing, concentration, and higher-level thinking skills. Cognitive therapists can work with you to regain some functioning, as well as offer strategies for compensating for any deficits. Many survivors rely on Social Security Disability Insurance (SSDI) benefits. SSDI allows you to work on a trial basis for up to nine months before terminating your benefits. SSDI also offers vocational rehabilitation programs to assist you with finding work suited to your special needs. If necessary, physical aids can be provided, as well as job-placement services. Contact your local Social Security office for more information.

APPENDIX L

Resources For Caregivers

Centers for Medicare and Medicaid Services

Medicaid pays for basic home healthcare and medical equipment. Medicaid may pay for homemaker, personal care, and other services that are not paid for by Medicare. For more information about what Medicaid covers for home healthcare in your state, call your state medical assistance office.

Related Links:

Medicare.gov:
The Official US Government Site for People with Medicare

CMS Regional Office Contact Information

"Caregiver Stress" at The Federal Government Source for Women's Health Information (PDF)

Eldercare Locator
A public service of the U.S. Administration on Aging, the Eldercare Locator can help you find local agencies, in every

US community, that can help older persons and their families' access home and community-based services like transportation, meals, home care, and caregiver support services.

Contact
Eldercare Locator, National Association of Area Agencies on Aging Toll Free: 800-677-1116 (Monday through Friday 9:00 am to 8:00 pm) E-mail: **eldercarelocator@n4a.org**

National Association of Area Agencies on Aging (n4a)
n4a's services for senior citizens who have restricted income include homemaker and home health aide services, transportation, home-delivered meals, chore and home repair as well as legal assistance. These government-funded services are often targeted to those most in need. While there are no income criteria for many services, sometimes you may have more service options if you can pay for private help. AAAs can direct you to other sources of help for older persons with limited incomes such as subsidized housing, food stamps, Supplemental Security Income, and Medicaid.

Contact
National Association of Area Agencies on Aging
1730 Rhode Island Ave, NW, Suite 1200
Washington, DC, 20036
Tel: 202-872-0888

Fax: 202-872-0057

Although the following organizations do not provide services for low-income individuals, they are an excellent source of information for caregivers:

Family Caregiver Alliance
180 Montgomery St, Ste 1100
San Francisco, CA 94104
Tel: 415-434-3388
Toll Free: 800-445-8106
Fax: 415-434-3508

National Family Caregivers Association
10400 Connecticut Avenue, Suite 500
Kensington, MD 20895-3944
Toll Free: 800-896-3650
Phone: 301-942-6430
Fax: 301-942-2302
E-mail: info@thefamilycaregiver.org